The Home Care Bible

*Tips of the Trade from the CEO
Perspective*

Written By

L. Smith-Pratt

Edited by Lisa M. Sundry

First Edition, 2018

DEDICATION

This book is dedicated to anyone, anywhere, who has opened, wanted to open, or will ever open a business that serves our community in two ways: by giving people jobs, and by ensuring that our incredibly valuable senior population has the choice to remain Independently at home.

FOREWORD

It was an August afternoon and I had just finished my shift. It was payday, so I trotted down to the office. At the time, I was a caregiver and didn't really know Lia personally. I also did not think she knew who I was. To my surprise, Lia was there that day, and the mood was a bit odd. Lia was firing the office manager, and that filled me with urgency. I needed this woman to know who I was and what I could offer her company.

I pretended not to notice what has happening and waited for the (former) office manager to walk out. I then took a deep breath and addressed Lia: "Hi, I overheard your conversation. It looks like you need a new office manager." Lia's quiet curiosity allowed me to continue. "I'll work for you for free for the next 30 days, just so you can see what I'm made of," I said, knowing full well that this was my big chance.

She was pleasantly surprised, and later I learned that it was because of my confidence and courage that she heard me out and gave me a chance. Lia hired me as her office manager. Later, I became her marketer.

After eight years of working for Lia, I approached her and shared my dream of starting my own home care agency. Her eyes filled with tears and so did mine. I was afraid of her reaction — would she chastise me and call me a traitor? I wasn't sure if I was more afraid of starting my own outfit or of leaving the place I'd grown so comfortable in.

But Lia wasn't angry, just sad to lose me. She quickly helped me come up with my company name and began giving me all the helpful advice you'll find in these pages. This advice has helped me launch and sustain a successful business that has been in steady growth since its inception. Lia wasn't a "wing clipper." Instead, she encouraged me to soar beyond my fear and uncertainty. She is my greatest supporter and ally.

Lia has mentored several of her past employees and encouraged them to start their own companies by offering advice and support. It was natural for her to grow into the role of franchisor, because this has been her greatest legacy: empowering and encouraging others to reach those dreams that feel far off and even unattainable.

In one of the last days I worked for her, she caught me sitting in her chair…in her office…and at her desk. I jokingly told her, "One day, I'll be the boss!" All told, I worked for Lia for eight years in two different companies, in all sorts of capacities. She was and continues to be a great inspiration and mentor.

Today, I *am* the boss. I sit at the chair and desk that Lia kindly gifted me, to remind myself of the potential this woman saw in me without fear or judgment—only with the noblest of intentions.

~*M. Hodges*
ACT Homecare, Co-Owner

The Home Care Bible

*Tips of the Trade
from the CEO Perspective*

ACKNOWLEDGMENTS

First and foremost, just as my ABS "dove of peace" logo indicates, I'd like to thank **God** for always getting our company through and taking us to new heights. There have been many influential people in my Home Care career, but I'd like to focus my thanks here on those who have made an impact on me in writing this book, specifically.

Kimberly Gerber of *iExcelerate Business Coaching* — you are first. Kimberly always wanted me to write a home care book, but I was too lazy; and truth be told I couldn't fathom having (making) the time to sit down and actually write a book while trying to DO home care! *Thank you for your belief in me at all times.* Even though things didn't work the way we planned, I am forever grateful to one of my first supervisors, mentors, and friend.

Next I'd like to thank **Kurt Buske** who literally bought into the dream and took the franchise system to a place where this book became necessary, who always has the courage to fight with me and the strength to have my back when I am afraid.

Thanks to **my team** at A Better Solution who believe in me and allow me to cheer *them* on and help them make things work; who "held down the fort" while I took the time to write this book: **Diana, Raquel, Dana, Jonah, Sabrina,** and the **outside team** that helps make it happen; **Brittany, Monique,** and the "Outcasts" (LOL) running our **Medicare Certified Home Health** — A Better Solution's "red headed stepchild."

I'd like to thank *the reason for this book* — my **first three franchise systems**, who have challenged me to create, assist and actually watch from the sidelines as someone else learns how to live their dreams. It is so much easier to actually DO something FOR someone than it is to wait and try to guide them in how to do it themselves. My "systems" are teaching me patience and how to play a supporting role, as well as the true meaning of, "Give a man a fish and he will eat for a day. Teach a man to fish and he will never go hungry."

"Thank You" specifically to my Rock Stars at this time, our first Franchise Partnership in Wichita, Kansas — **Gus and Amy** — who first had faith in me and our concept; and to **Dave and Brett**, who are continuing to learn the ropes (and who will probably create the need for another book, *Home Care Bible II — The Sequel!*), as well as the other systems that have come on since.

Special thanks to **Ruth Herrera Buske**, who takes the time to read through my work, and all of the things I put out, who makes me sound smarter than I am, and keeps me from rushing the process. She is the best personal assistant ever! (Another inside joke—she is really a **Public Relations Manager**, but I am very High Maintenance, and she is patient with me.)

And of course, thank you to my very own "**Dragon Lady**" **Lisa Sundry, my book editor,** who gently prods me to explain myself in a manner that everyone can understand, and makes sense out of the madness and raw information I write.

There are things missing from this book, but I had to stop somewhere, because Home Care and business building are topics that I could talk about all day, every day. They are my passion, and watching others grow is where I find my deepest joy.

So feel free to take and keep notes on the back pages of this book, and email me with any questions you may have. I hope you enjoy your Journey Through Home Care, and that your career path is filled with deep appreciation and financial success.

CONTENTS

INTRODUCTION

A Better Solution In Home Care, Inc. ("ABS") is a brand and a company culture that is Client and Caregiver driven — meaning, unless you follow some very simple steps, your agency will not grow to the same level of success as our other Franchise Partners who follow our Client-Centric Model, even though your agency carries the ABS name. Our development team can sell you a Brand, but they cannot be there while you make the daily decisions that truly create your company culture, which is the key to assuring your environment will be rich in success, with fulfillment from both the clients and caregivers. That is what will truly determine your leading role in the industry. This Guide will tell you not just the HOW of things (you have our manuals to do that), it will tell you the WHY of things, and that knowledge will assist you greatly as you build and grow.

Owning a Home Care/Senior Care agency is filled with incredible highs...and incredible moments of doubt. A Better Solution In Home Care, Inc. calls itself a Home Care Agency — not a *senior care agency*. Many people are confused by the definitions and terms in our industry, but ABS does all types of care, and one of them just happens to be senior care. In addition, many of the "types" or revenue streams we provide have absolutely nothing to do with a home setting. But perception is everything, and for many years *caregivers* were for seniors and *nurses* were for hospitals. Not today. Our scope of practice has widened to include so many different aspects of care, from mentally disabled children, both with respite and in schools, to placing seniors in assisted living communities all over the county, and both of these are very lucrative streams of income, but neither have anything to do with the old perception of Senior Care. Call it what you wish—this book is specifically designed for our Franchise Partners to give further insight and knowledge into the animal that is your Home Care Agency. ~L. Smith-Pratt

CHAPTER 1
THE CHICKEN OR THE EGG

(Caregivers Before Clients)

Many people wonder, and we are often asked, "What comes first—the 'Chicken' or the 'Egg'?"

The answer is…Caregivers before Clients. And your Caregiver Roster is your nest of Eggs.

It seems counterintuitive to begin hiring caregivers before you have any clients to place them with. But the hiring of caregivers is a slower, more methodical process, and actually one of the more *fun* aspects of owning a home care business. A Better Solution In Home Care, Inc. has what we like to call a *Caregiver Roster*; which is no more than a list of caregivers who we have cleared to work for our clients. The trick is to find the RIGHT caregiver for each client.

In the beginning, it takes a few tries. And because of that, you need to have many caregivers available before you ever get that first client. Hiring is a much longer process (see Chapters 2 through 4) and many of the caregivers are not actually sitting around waiting for your call—many of them apply for a variety of home care jobs with several agencies and may likely be unavailable even if you call them the next day for a shift.

On top of that, when starting your agency, the majority of first referrals are going to be emergency referrals that no one else wants. So you will spend much less time frustrated if you have 15 to 25 caregivers to call and ask to take your open shifts.

"...The hiring of caregivers is a slower, more methodical process, and actually one of the more fun aspects of owning a home care business."

Many CEO's will stop after hiring five or six caregivers because they begin to feel "guilty" about not having work for them, or they fall into the trap of forgetting that we start with the egg—because we never know when the chicken will come along.

Regardless, fill your roster, have at least 25 caregivers *you have met personally* and that have been cleared through your system to work. If you don't, you will either end up taking care of clients yourself, hiring someone off the street or trying to place friends and family with clients—or worse yet—turning down clients all together, which is the death of a new agency.

So remember this chapter.

✔ **Hire ongoing—always hire.** Don't stop! For many

reasons, caregivers are the lifeblood of your home care agency, and out of every five you hire, usually only one will work out.

No matter WHAT they tell you:

✔ **You need to have a roster full so you have choices (good ones) for your clients when they need your services.** Caregivers are working for multiple agencies, going to school, doing many things that will render them unavailable for the exact hours and days you may need them.

> *"Hire ongoing—always hire.*
> *Don't stop!"*

✔ **Caregivers have potential value for many other aspects of your home care agency down the road.** A polished and professional caregiver may be your next Jr. Marketing person, Care Manager, or Staffing/Administrative Assistant, so keep hiring.

Bottom line: The general rule is 25 caregivers on your roster before you even take one case, and three caregivers for every case you have. Remember, for every five you hire, four will fall off, and when they do, take them off of your roster and continually replenish with good, strong caregivers as you move forward.

The Home Care Bible

CHAPTER 2
THE EGG

(Hiring Caregivers & Where To Find Them)

This is one of the most frequently asked questions during our initial phone conversations with prospective Franchisees: *How do you find caregivers?* Which, if you are in the industry, you know there is no shortage of people willing to be hired to become caregivers. There is, however, a process of elimination of those that apply and get interviewed, and those that actually want work consistently, who are good with all types of clients, are neat and professional in manner, and that will actually *stay* with your agency on a long term basis.

> *"Time is valuable as a CEO. You don't have much of it, so don't waste it. Work Smarter, Not Harder."*

Suffice it to say, "caregivers" are everywhere! But the process you choose to hire them may take many different forms. Our corporate office has continual ads

in *Indeed* (which is the hot resume source right now —
may be another in your area); it has taken over for
Craigslist or the Pennysaver. We run a paid ad through
Indeed's website. I do like to run one through
Craigslist as well, as it is relatively inexpensive ($35 in
San Diego). You may also post on your Facebook or
LinkedIn page.

As we have grown, we have begun active
"recruitment" at Nursing or CNA schools to get
caregivers from those sources.

Some Tips of the Trade:

1. Always Schedule Two Interviews At a Time

If you do not have an office with open recruitment
hours, and are working from a schedule, you will find
that one out of three applicants never show up, and if
you have set aside time, you don't want it wasted. If
they all show up, perfect; they can complete the
applications while you conduct the individual
interviews. But more than likely only one will show
up — and he or she won't be the one with the perfect
resume!

So schedule several interviews at a time, even if you
are working from an office or at a Starbucks — unless
you want to sit there all day because no one showed
up at 9 a.m. and 11 a.m., but you have another one
scheduled for 2 p.m. Set up the interviews or
applicants 10 minutes apart all day long.

2. Always lead with, "What are you currently doing?"

The Roster Filler: If someone is currently working full-time, they are not available to you, but they might be a great "Roster Filler"—someone who may work 2-3 days for you in a pinch, or eventually come on board full-time later if you pay more competitively than the other guys.

The Roster Filler should have already been fingerprinted and registered (depending on your state requirements) and be able to immediately go into orientation with you and ready to work. I like Roster Fillers—I don't feel guilty when I don't have work for them, they tend to look professional, and if I can work around their other schedule, they usually are reliable and know what they are doing.

3. Your second question should always be, "Are you cleared to work?"

✔ **State Clearance & Tracking:** Your state will have caregiver requirements. If they don't, then skip this question. If they do, how far along is your applicant in the process? And does he/she expect or need your help? In the beginning, I do not provide help—I have no case for them yet, so I am not willing to spend money on a caregiver I may or may not need. *But also, I need to assess how much time is needed to TRACK your progress on getting everything you need to be available for immediate work.*

✔ **ABS does not recommend you track people longer than one week.** For example, if they interview but need fingerprinting, TB testing, but already have a registration card, you give them 5 business days to get everything back to you—and you let them know they will have to REAPPLY in 7 days if they do not have the documentation.

✔ **Let them know that, after 7 days, if they do not bring the clearances back—you will shred the application.** What this protocol does for you: It means less useless paperwork with sensitive information laying around—and you will not be tempted to call them when you are in a jam.

"I like Roster Fillers—I don't feel guilty when I don't have work for them, they tend to look professional, and if I can work around their other schedule, they usually are reliable and know what they are doing."

4. Presentation—Do They Look The Part?

Bottom line: There must be a balance between having standards for professional appearance and demeanor & judging too harshly.

✔ **Are your applicants neatly dressed?** Do they have tattoos that are offensive or will be difficult to cover? Are they wearing scrubs already? Do they have wild, blue hair? Missing teeth? Poor grammar or don't speak clearly? Are they rude or angry looking? Confrontational or defensive? Secretive or reeking of alcohol? Do they have four kids with them? Or, are they kind, clean, willing to answer questions thoroughly (without going on and on) and calm? Professional and well-groomed? Did they take the time to dress nicely for the interview? However they show up to meet you is how they will show up eventually to a client's location.

✔ **Do they have the knowledge that you need?** ABS has application questionnaires available for you to follow in our Franchise Portal, so you will be able — even without any prior experience of your own — to find out if the applicants "know their stuff." If they do, you may need to overlook some of the outside things, because a good caregiver comes in many different forms, colors, personalities, and attitudes.

✔ **Don't judge too harshly. Remember: Caregivers come in all shapes, sizes, colors, and personalities**. At first, newer owners begin this process like they were hiring an office staff person. They interview for long periods of time (30-45 minutes). They have a "feeling" about an applicant because they don't *appear* as the owner expected. As new owners, we seem to think that we need to establish an "employer-employee" relationship, or that we are going to find out deep, dark secrets that will tip us off to good and bad caregivers.

Well, newsflash: You won't. You don't even have immediate work available yet, so you are simply looking for a "type" at this point.

✔ **What to prioritize, then?** The answer is — it depends. You must weigh the strengths and weaknesses one applicant at a time. A caregiver who inspires confidence and comfort, a caregiver with an upbeat personality is better than a skilled, cranky person who is sharply dressed. A caregiver who laughs easily, has questions for you, or who knows his/her skill set, is great. An arrogant know-it-all is not.

"...Schedule several interviews at a time, even if you are working from an office or at a Starbucks—unless you want to sit there all day because no one showed up."

5. State your expectations clearly: "I am putting together a roster of great caregivers so I can begin my Home Care service."

✔ **Let them know that you are new and will be calling for new positions, and that they should be ready to take on the whole case if they are available.** Let them know you will be holding an orientation the following week—for one-to-five hours (depending on your state's requirements). *This will show you if they will come back.*

✔ **Tell them that, as a new agency, you need exceptional people with uniforms and a professional appearance, as well as great personalities.** Caregivers need to know—clearly—your expectation in this regard. Like so many positions, this one deals with clients/customers—so customer service is key. Difficult situations are what your caregivers are walking into, so loud or aggressive types don't work in home care.

✔ **Do they show up?** Your orientation is really your second chance to see *who* shows up and *how* they show up, so don't waste too much time yapping (interviewing) about yourself and the company expectations in your first interview. They may never show up again. Time is valuable as a CEO. You don't have much of it, so don't waste it. Work Smarter, Not Harder.

"A caregiver who laughs easily, has questions for you, or who knows his/her skill set, is great. An arrogant know-it-all is not."

6. The Initial Questions to Ask Them — and Why

✔ **Where do you currently work?** This will tell you what agencies are usually slow—because working caregivers don't have the time to interview.

✔ **How much is your current pay?** Some caregivers will hedge a little on this one, but if they have other agencies listed on their application, ask them. It lets you know the industry standard for pay rates.

✔ **Why are you looking for work?** This is an *open-ended question* that will tell you more about the caregiver in general, what he/she has been or is currently doing, and how amiable he/she really is.

✔ **What do you <u>like</u> about your current work place**?

Pro Tip: If it is home care, you can take tips of the trade from their response, and find out how you can incorporate those things into *your* agency.

✔ **What <u>don't</u> you like about your agency?** This is where you can find out if the caregiver is a *Company Basher*: "They never pay, they are going bankrupt, they don't ever have work, my clients are too hard, it's too far, I'm underappreciated," and on and on.

It is nice to take a few nuggets from this, but also really listen—because one day he/she may be saying the same things to someone else about *you*, and it may even be to one of your clients.

> *"Difficult situations are what your caregivers are walking into, so loud or aggressive types don't work in home care."*

We like to hear, "They don't have work currently," or, "I don't have enough hours."

Anything else, put a note in your system to remember what this caregiver needs, especially when he/she says any of the following: "They don't give good instruction," "They never check on the client," "They send me too far," "The staffers/boss/office staff are short tempered, rude," "My pay is always wrong," or, "They promised me one rate and paid another."

Bottom Line: If you hear, "They have all hard clients," or, "They asked me to do too much"—stay aware of what he/she is truly saying, and how this caregiver may be a problem for you later.

7. Closing the Interview

✔ **Ask a few "horizon" questions:**

~What are you hoping to find in your new position?

~What would your presence *add* to the company you work for?

✔ **Verify contact information.** This one may seem obvious, but make sure you have their correct, current contact information (phone, email, mailing address).

Pro Tip: When you are interviewing, you should have each interviewee's application/resume in a manila file folder, so you can place it on your desk to refer to.

Once the interview is over, hand it to your receptionist to begin checking references, or leave it on the table — *covered* — while you hold the other interviews.

The Home Care Bible

CHAPTER 3
ORIENTATION

(What is it and why do it?)

There are very few states left who do not have a licensure law for home care, and some of them, like California, include regulations for caregiving and staff members as well. So, at times, orientation—its duration and content—will be predetermined by the state in which you open your agency, and for other states it will not be a requirement.

Whether or not it is a legal requirement, our Franchise Partners are taught and expected to hold a 2-Hour Orientation for every caregiver and staff member they hire. The reason for this is twofold: Away from the formal interview process, there are many things you can determine about a person in an informal "orientation" setting—how they speak, how they listen, *and whether or not they show up.*

Depending on your state labor laws, you may hold an orientation for under two hours, and if that is a basis for hiring, you may or may not be required to pay a wage for it. If you do, we recommend having a sign in sheet and paying this at your state or city minimum wage.

"...There are many things you can determine about a person in an informal 'orientation' setting—how they speak, how they listen, and whether or not they show up."

No matter what the circumstances, there are several things that need to be conveyed at your orientation for the ABS brand and culture to be effective within your agency:

1. The Basics: What You Need to Know

✔ **How many do I schedule?** If you have the space in your headquarters, then 6-10 applicants per orientation is appropriate. But if you are starting out as a home-based agency, you should rent a conference room, or other room space close by, and put as many caregivers in there as you can fit. We highly recommend you have an orientation every week until you have a roster of 25-30. Thereafter, you can schedule them every two weeks.

✔ **Alert them on the front end!** Tell every person you interview WHEN and WHERE your next orientation will be so they are not waiting for a call or lost in the shuffle. Many will obtain employment before you get around to orientation (yes, that quickly), and some, though hired elsewhere, will attend anyway if they already know when it is.

✔ **Are they on time?**

Pro Tip: Call the day before, leaving messages — reminding "New Hires" of the upcoming orientation, so there is no reason to arrive more than five minutes late. And if they do arrive late, did they call *en route*?

✔ **Can you create a synergy?** Caregivers have opinions and questions, and this is the time when you want them to talk. You are asking things like, "Who has worked in home care before?" "Who is willing to drive 25 miles for full-time work?" Etc.

You want them laughing and enjoying working together with you.

As the leader in the agency, you are taking the first steps to creating a loyalty to you and to your agency, which will go farther than the money you pay, or the jobs you offer. A loyal caregiver will always do his/her best, because they are not working for the client — they are working for YOU.

"Caregivers have opinions and questions, and this is the time when you want them to talk."

✔ **Pick out, focus on and flag your favorites — they will be client favorites as well.** Place a star by their names after orientation, they are the ones you want to call first. Especially place a star if you are the one holding the orientation but not staffing your own cases, because there WILL be a communication breakdown between you and your staffers.

Pro Tip: Help your staffers to help you. The reality is that, from the staffers' perspective, these are names on a pile of paper *EVEN IF* they have interviewed some of these new hires. Staffers forget, they are busy, they are constantly interrupted throughout the day.

So you need to communicate to them WHO represents your "Ideal" caregivers best suited to represent your agency. Otherwise you are just a talking head — your staffers may like and know you, but you have NOT communicated and effectively utilized your orientation process to strengthen your caregiver knowledge base and create a better reputation.

Clients like who we like. Those are your front runners and you want to place them quickly. So place a star and put a little notation in their file that reads something like:

"Great appearance!"
"Asked great questions."
"USE HER!" is what I like to say!

> *"We highly recommend you have an orientation every week until you have a roster of 25-30 and then you can schedule them every two weeks."*

✔ **Don't over-talk or complicate the orientation by getting too off-topic.** Caregivers get bored, as do clients and their families. *Use this time as practice for reading people and catching the signs*, and changing course and direction. You will also need this skill as you assess clients in order to pick out non-verbal clues that you are selling too hard, or talking too long without listening.

2. Communicate Your Expectations, Describe Your Brand & Set the Bar NOW

Other than state requirements, below are some of the things your caregivers must know and understand.

These are just a FEW:

✔ **Be on time.** If you are constantly late you, will be removed from our roster. We are responsible both financially and ethically for a block of time, and if something occurs during that time—whether we are there or not—we can be held liable. So be on time, and don't change hours or days without company notification.

✔ **Be kind and courteous** to all who come to the door and enter the home, and especially to our clients.

✔ **Never leave a client alone.** Do not leave the room to use your phone, "run home for a minute," or go to your car. *If there is an emergency, call the office and let US replace you.*

✔ **Show up professionally.** We are not our clients' friends. We are caregivers in the caregiving profession, and as such, we wear clean, pressed scrubs, close-toed shoes, no facial piercings or long nails.

✔ **Do not get involved in family matters.** You are not

family, and you will be the first to go when they make up, or learn of your opinions. So try to keep talk light and listen more than you speak.

✔ **Do not take anything from the home.** This should be self-explanatory. If a client wants to give a gift, it should be done in writing and submitted to the office.

✔ **Do not bring anything or anyone IN the home.** No children, cousins with a cleaning service, husbands, pets, etc. Our liability insurance does not cover those who are not employees.

✔ **Do not riffle through clients' belongings.** Even when putting away laundry, make sure the client is in the room. If things are missing, you have to be above reproach.

✔ **Report, Report, Report** — submitted in writing to the office — if something happens to the client; a fall, confusion, change in behavior or need.

✔ **Remember who you work for** — "The Agency" — not the client — so do not solicit them for more work, go by the house on non-working hours, call them and change the schedule, "borrow things" or even loan things. **Stay professional.**

✔ **Have fun!** *Create an environment of happiness and calm.* Make YOUR time with the client be the best time of their day. Caregivers touch lives, and every time should be a wonderful experience for the person they care for.

✔ **Keep negativity out of the home.** Do not discuss your problems, your children, your spouse, etc. They are paying clients, not therapists or counselors. Even when they ask: "Everything is fine," is an appropriate answer.

✔ **Never change your own schedule.** Changing your own schedule puts the client and the agency at risk, because the client has contracted for a set amount of days and hours, and if something occurs during those hours we are liable.

"A loyal caregiver will always do his/her best, because they are not working for the client—they are working for YOU."

The Home Care Bible

CHAPTER 4
CAREGIVER QUALITIES
~ THE THREE "R's" ~

Reliable, Responsible & Respectful

1. Caregiver Kindness

If this were a clothing store, the caregivers would be your clothing. If we were a restaurant, the caregivers would be your food. So quality counts, but just as you wouldn't throw away every potato that has a blemish or a pair of pants that is a color you don't like, don't *overthink* your caregivers. The most important things about them you will truly not know until they actually work.

I have had many Franchise Partners say they want "perfect" caregivers, and they want to check every application and do every interview themselves. That is great, if you have a marketer doing the other part of your work, but remember—the best caregiver shows up on time, is respectful, professional and anticipates the client's needs. These things you won't find out until you give them an actual client.

Pro Tip: Caregivers are masters at the interview. They deal with people for a profession, so some of your worst caregivers are the ones that novice owners like the most: They have the best excuses for being late, not showing up, or leaving early. The excuses just keep rolling in, and you buy into them one by one.

What I have learned many times is that my very best caregivers are the ones that I rarely see or speak with — they call in, get an assignment, and they are Reliable, Responsible and Respectful (the three R's).

"The best caregiver shows up on time, is respectful, professional and anticipates the client's needs. These things you won't find out until you give them an actual client."

2. The Three R's. In order to get the full time clients and the best rate of pay, your caregivers should be:

✔ **Reliable** — Meaning, the caregiver not only arrives early, he/she has scoped out the client's home and mapped out transportation directions the day before; that the caregiver is *consistently* reliable; takes ownership over that client and what they need and what they want; that the Agency can *rely* upon them to report any problems or occurrences with the client; and that the caregiver can be counted on by the family.

✔ **Responsible** — With everyone's things and care. The caregiver can be relied upon not to take things or create unnecessary conflict — within the client's home, or the agency. Shows that they can be trusted with anything the client throws at them and can adapt to any changes in situation; that his/her Responses are the same as the Agency's Core Values and they can be counted on for that.

✔ **Respectful** — Of their teammates, their client, the client's family, and the office staff. This client is vulnerable and in a weakened state; they are paying for the agency to provide them with kind and loving care. When you have a wonderful caregiver who is respectful of the client and their family, their privacy, their things, and their feelings, you have a client that feels safe in his or her home.

Bottom Line: Respect is something that cannot be taught. Caregivers either have it or they don't. So if you have a caregiver that will lose his/her temper with you or the office staff, they will likely do the same with clients, family, or even referral sources. Don't take that chance.

"What I have learned many times is that my very best caregivers are the ones that I rarely see or speak with, they call in, get an assignment, and they are Reliable, Responsible and Respectful (the three R's)."

The Home Care Bible

CHAPTER 5
THE CHICKEN

(Clients: Who are they?)

Before you go searching for clients, you need to know who they are. In our Training System, you will go through "Pitch Your Niche," which is where we work with you to find YOUR personal passion, coupled with your territory's specific care needs that are not being met, and help you to develop a marketing campaign around that—but first things first: *Who are they, these Mysterious Clients?*

We spend so much time as new owners worrying about our caregivers' qualities that we forget that our clients come in a range of sizes, shapes, needs, personalities, expectations, and looks. There is no "typical client." The client you probably see in your mind is the sweet, 80-year-old lady who is a little forgetful and maybe has to be watched so she doesn't give all of her money to the Canadian Lottery, or who is walking with a cane and just needs a little help.

"Here are the car keys, we need to go to the

store.' 'I don't think I need you tomorrow, so don't come,' or 'I am fine now, you can leave.' All of these are not acceptable, and can be dangerous."

A Better Solution does not have "Senior Care" as a part of our name because, in the last (at the time of writing) 18 years, we have found that clients for our Franchise system come in all ages, shapes and sizes—from special needs children to perfectly fine middle aged adults getting plastic surgery, to facilities that we provide staffing support to. So let's go through the specifics of some of these clients.

Who Are They? The different types of clients you will encounter:

1. Your Typical Senior

Diagnosis, dementia, forgetfulness, broken hip, transportation needs, just plain loneliness. Less and less are we finding the "Companion Cases," where the clients just need company to be there and do the little things for them.

With all of the changes to the insurance industry and minimum wage requirements, care has become too expensive for many of those who desperately need it, or who would have in the past utilized it more often. Seniors come from an era where things were much less expensive, so someone who can otherwise barely walk will suddenly dance a jig when they get your first bill, and either cut hours or quit service altogether.

A lot of these clients come from adult children who do not have the time to help out in the home. These clients are lonely, no matter what the medical condition is, and they are the ones usually very easy to fall in love with. Seniors can be cranky, feisty, irritable — or sweet, kind, and easygoing, but either way, these are the clients we expected and visualized when we started our agency.

Pro Tip: These are also the clients that need your highest level of caregivers, with the three R's. Why? *Because they are usually home alone.* If your caregiver does not show up, many times you will not know until it is too late. So if you don't have a **Reliable**, **Responsible** and **Respectful** person in the home, you can place someone's safety in very real danger — truly — and this is not acceptable, and will earn you a terrible reputation.

> *"(T)he caregiver has to be respectful and understand that the Primary Caregiver (the family member in the house) is also the 'boss.' … The caregiver you assign will need to be able to hold their tongue and just patiently listen."*

2. Respite Care

Typically, this can be either older adults being cared for by adult children or special needs children being cared for by parents. Either way, the money for care comes from either grants or government programs, and these clients differ from the seniors in that *they have an advocate in the home to watch out for them and also to oversee the care they receive.*

In both instances under this category, the actual client is probably easier to please than the person taking care of them—*so they both become your client.* The most important qualities your caregiver will need here are **Reliability** (there is someone else depending on the Respite) and **Respect**.

The adult child and or the parents can be very high strung and detailed when giving instructions to the caregiver, as well as terribly picky about the caregiver you send. So the caregiver has to be respectful and understand that the Primary Caregiver (the family member in the house) is also the "boss."

Pro Tip: The caregiver you assign will need to be able to hold their tongue and just patiently listen. *All the time.*

3. Perfectly Fine, Outpatient Type Surgeries

This is another category of high maintenance clients, due to the fact that they are not incapacitated in any way except for the post-surgery recovery period.

For these clients you are looking for your **Responsible** caregivers, as these clients tend to overstep the bounds of the client-caregiver relationship—"Here is my ATM card. Go pull some money out to grocery shop." "Here are the car keys, we need to go to the store." "I don't think I need you tomorrow, so don't come," or "I am fine now, you can leave." All of these are not acceptable, and can be dangerous.

These clients are also the ones that need a more presentable caregiver — the mental picture of a "Nurse" is firmly in their mind, and you need to get close to that image.

Pro Tip: You also need to be sure to get a *preference sheet* on these clients — they are your short term, but high dollar clients. *They are your word of mouth referrals,* and they are very particular. A great caregiver placed here can buy you another week of service and a bad caregiver will have your reputation with the doctor or clinic tanked.

"The client you probably see in your mind is the sweet, 80-year-old lady who is a little forgetful and maybe has to be watched so she doesn't give all of her money to the Canadian Lottery, or who is walking with a cane and just needs a little help."

4. Registry/Facility Staffing, a.k.a. Shift Work

This is where you are going for "shift work," so it is a numbers game and not a "perfect match" need. Your caregiver *look* and *feel* matters less. Here it is all about **Reliability**. You need **three** caregivers who will show up and work on shifts. *If they are not on time you will look bad, and if they are unskilled you will look bad.*

These are your low margin, high volume, short term clients. Your client here is the staffing counterpart in your facility, as well as the HR department, to ensure that all of the paperwork is correct. Your client is the facility and that makes it much easier to staff.

CHAPTER 6
MARKETING

(How do I get clients?)

The second and most important question! And where the work comes in: "The Chicken."

So you have been told that Clients are everywhere — Baby Boomers are getting older, and they are in the grocery store and they are your next door neighbors. Once you own a home care company, suddenly potential seems to be everywhere, and you are all over the place looking for those clients!

We frequently get asked questions like: *Should I go to this health fair? Should I advertise on the grocery store receipts? Should I put money into this Marketing Strategy? Should I go to that seminar? This guy's great over here, should I spend money on his program?*

Well, this is your chapter!

With A Better Solution Franchise, we have several different consultants we pay to train you in your first two weeks, in a classroom setting of practicum, and then with actual procedural training. Where ABS provides two weeks of training, most franchises offer only one week. Why did we change? Because, as much as we try to *build* your confidence, the only way we feel that can happen is if you truly ARE confident in your knowledge and skill set.

"Marketing is the sales process that occurs when you meet those that actually refer to you and those that need you."

We noticed some of our newer franchise partners reaching out and attending overly expensive marketing seminars — assuming there was a "secret" to sell services and being successful and, as a result, spending money unnecessarily.

The most important element after acquiring caregivers is knowing *how and where to get clients* — they are your revenue, and a business cannot survive without it. Attending marketing seminars is not the answer, so in this comprehensive chapter, we will go through all of the tips, skill sets and approaches that we have trained you in, but we will go into a little more detail to help you understand the WHY of what we recommend.

1. Understanding Marketing Principles Specific to Home Care

✔ **Branding.** *Branding* is the practice of creating a name, symbol, logo or design that differentiates your service from others. Here at corporate (ABS), we have created the logo, contracts, training materials for staff and all marketing collateral for you. We have established the foundational aspects for you—like the mission statement, list of core values, company benefits and features, as well as your business model. Everything is uniform. That is your *brand*.

✔ **Marketing.** *Marketing* in home care is often referred to as "business-to-business sales." This type of marketing is the process that occurs when you meet those who will actually refer to you, and those that will actually need your services. This is the "boots on the ground" approach: going to hospitals, skilled nursing facilities, assisted livings and so on. We will go through some examples of both in this chapter.

Here is what you need to know and implement in order to successfully market for new clients:

2. Ground Zero for Marketing: Know Your Biggest Mistakes—*Before* You Make Them

✔ **"I can Health Fair my way into success!"** Health fairs are BRANDING opportunities, not marketing. They are branding your agency in the community, getting your name known by way of promotion. Only. And, *it is definitely one of the biggest and most prevalent mistakes I see new owners make.*

It is an unfortunate waste of time, energy and money. It is great for the lazy marketer, however—to stand and give away your pens and brochures, maybe even bags, or a $25-$100 gift for a "raffle" to all the people who walk by and say hello.

"Our type of business requires people to be sick, and rarely do you find sick people wandering through the aisle of a health fair picking up pens."

Well, common sense dictates, if they are *walking*, they don't need care. And on the off chance that they "Know Someone," you will have spent 30 minutes talking that could have been spent in a hospital or nursing facility.

We recommend our Franchise Partners pick ONE system to support. What we have done is choose one large hospital system, and we support everything they do. Our goal is to slowly brand our name with theirs.

✔ **Community Health Fairs vs. Exhibits.** The "Health Fairs" I do attend cost so much money that I had to wait until I'd been in business for over 10 years before I could afford them! **And the term here is "Exhibit" — not "Health Fair."**

These exhibits are at conferences where referral sources gather (i.e. PFAC — Professional Fiduciary and Conservators; CALA — California Assisted Living Association), and they are upwards of $2,000, but I can now *Brand* on a higher level. (These exhibits are more for branding than marketing.)

The problem with "community" health fairs is they cost anywhere from Free to $100, and they are usually promoting the community they are in — or the agency putting it together. The relationships you will make at these fairs are with other vendors doing the same thing as you: sitting at a booth trying to get their name out there.

The vendors who sell products have the greatest success at these fairs. Community-based health fairs are a great place for widgets and merchandise because people can shop and conclude transactions. Our type of business is service-based and requires people to be sick, and rarely do you find sick people wandering through the aisle of a health fair picking up pens.

"We recommend our Franchise Partners pick ONE system to support. What we have done is choose one large hospital system, and we support everything they do. Our goal is to slowly brand our name with theirs."

✔ **"I can advertise my way to success**." Not on your budget you can't! It is easy to get out of control with publication advertising, too. I have been traveling on an airplane and seen an ad for a home care franchise in the airline magazine (you know, the one in the pocket you pick up when you forgot *your* magazine, the one that has articles on all of the exotic places you will never visit?) and I thought to myself as I read that ad, "Never in my life have I been flying somewhere and thought about buying a Home Care Franchise!"

The numbers were inflated, it was full of information, and I am sure it cost thousands to place that ad due to the National Reach.

"Every territory has referral potential, no matter what they say. You have to find the

right person. And higher end clients don't necessarily come from higher end communities, they come from medical need."

By the same token, I have had my marketers run to me in fear saying, "I was just at the grocery store and Company X has its logo on the coupon part of the receipt! Oh, no! Can we do this? Please? It is only $1 per receipt!"

You mean the part of the receipt I throw away after I shop? That part? With one dollar off milk or cookies, or whatever else I have already purchased? No. I would do better spending $250-$700 on pens and brochures and actually *marketing*!

✔ **"I can join networking groups and 'get to know people.'"** I am on the board for the state association, and I have been chair for our regional council, and many of my marketers have held positions on local networking groups and on business networking sites that cost anywhere from $25 a meeting to thousands a year.

What I can tell you from this experience is that these interactions are not very helpful from a marketing standpoint. Why? Because YOU will be the ONLY business of your type in the group! That is too much money and time spent for a "maybe" referral.

Traditional methods don't work in home care. We are in a business that is only needed when people are in trouble, so volume referrals don't come from your community.

I see newer agencies trying to latch onto other marketers and owners. "Let's get together!" they say to me. "Why?" I think. They need mentors – not networking with competitors. (See Chapter 14 on Mentors.)

Pro Tip: New agency owners TALK, TALK, TALK. Don't do that. Loose lips give out too much information and do not create mutually beneficial business relationships. "Where do you do your business?" and, "Have you worked with this or that hospital?" Not yet – but I will DEFINITELY go over there now. There *are* exceptions. **But I believe networking groups are to be generally used as a promotional tool to *legitimize* your agency once you are confident enough to act like you have some sense.**

Larger agencies are NOT at networking groups. Why? Because they are BUSY MARKETING! There truly may be enough business to go around, but my motto is, if *you* are *getting* clients – then *I* am *losing* clients, so I am fiercely competitive.

> *"I believe networking groups are to be generally used as a tool to legitimize your agency once you are confident enough to act like you have some sense."*

Every so often I will click with someone in our industry and I may test the "friendship" waters. Sometimes it works, and sometimes it doesn't. I have found it easier when I have no agenda, so I (as the Owner), or Kurt (as the President) can make connections because we vibrate at a higher level than your traditional marketer, and usually have a better sense of who to talk to, as we don't have a lot of time outside of operations to spend with colleagues within the industry unless the relationships are mutually beneficial.

✔ **I recommend only going to networking groups when you want to check the pulse**.

~When business is good, stop in and say hello.

~When business is bad, check in and see what your colleagues are doing.

~Lunches? I do them when I am marketing, to create a deeper relationship, and sometimes I actually find a few friends, but I don't ask friends for business, so lunches for me can be counter-productive.

We tend to befriend those at higher levels than we are, and as you grow it will be easier, and you will look more to "Mentors" than "Colleagues." Mentors you watch but don't spend much time with.

✔ **"I can 'friend' my way to success."** This is, you guessed it, another funny one. This one *does work* but it takes forever! I still get sucked into this. Someone is the Director of Marketing for a hospice. Impressive, right? Whoo hooo! They want to have lunch with me! We go...I buy...we talk...about kids, life, other people; and now we are friends! Yaaayyy.

Weeks pass and I never hear from them. I see them and, whoo hooo, we have lunch again! We are getting somewhere now! She/he tells me we will exchange referrals — Yes, yes. I send him/her one — whoo hooo — and if they are savvy at this game, they will now send you a client *you cannot service* but which does get your hopes up! It is working! You send them a few more. WOW — this is awesome!

Unless you work for me, this could go on for YEARS.

> *"If you want to cross-refer be upfront: Directly tell people, 'I will refer to you, but if you don't refer back, I am moving on to the next guy.'"*

I have watched my marketers place people in Assisted Livings over and over again for a "Gift Card," when placement agencies (and we are one as well) are getting THOUSANDS for their placement.

But we are FRIENDS and I am going to get this reciprocated…right?

I have watched my marketers send Home Health Referrals over and over to agencies who have sent us ***two*** clients. Now, as the Owner I can stop this — by making my marketers aware of the actual numbers. But if you fall into this trap as an owner, the only thing that will get you out of this habit will be boredom with the chit chat.

A true friendship is based on love and respect, and most (if not all) of the time, in my industry-related friendships — although business is discussed — referrals may never come up, because we are fierce competitors and business is secondary. When I do get a referral from a friend, I treat it with kid gloves because I feel responsible, and I owe it to them, and honestly — at this juncture — it isn't worth the stress.

So keep things professional. If you want to *cross-refer* be upfront: Directly tell people, "I will refer to you, but if you don't refer back, I am moving on to the next guy." For your own sake, don't mix business with friendships in the industry, as it can ruin both, especially if you are looking to gain business out of the relationship. That is a *colleague* not *a friend*.

> *"For your own sake, don't mix business with friendships in the industry, as it can ruin both."*

✔ **"The territory I am in is not good enough."** Marketers make this declaration all the time, and new owners are even funnier — they want to go to the more upscale areas: "People have money in (insert wealthy area of your town here). I need to market there!" Even though their territory is (insert NON-wealthy area in your town!).

"I mean, it has been 30 days and I haven't gotten a bite, so I am going over *there* now." Unfortunately, rich areas are being brokered by SKILLED marketing personnel — which, if you haven't gotten anything out of your own territory in 30 days — common sense says you are not one.

Now, 18 years later, if I focus and spend two weeks somewhere, I am sure to get a referral. Why? **Because**

I don't deviate from my focus. Every territory has referral potential, no matter what they say. You have to find the right person. And higher end clients don't necessarily come from higher end communities, they come from medical need.

For example, if I have a "rich" area person with Alzheimer's, their kids are a little more savvy and a little more attached to mom or dad's money. They tend to oversee like crazy and start with very low hours. The case will grow, but they are picky, so by the time it does, if you have not staffed it well, it will go to another agency (see Chapter 9 — Staffing).

> *"(R)ich areas are being brokered by SKILLED marketing personnel—which, if you haven't gotten anything out of your own territory in 30 days—common sense says you are not one."*

Conversely, in, say, an area of lower income — for us it's Kearney Mesa (there are at least 10 hospices, home health agencies, skilled nursing facilities, etc.) — I may get lower end clients but they are less likely to have children overseeing them, and they are in crisis, so the care is short term but high hours. I may have 1-3 hospice cases that only last a week but they are all 24-hour and $23 per hour. *More bang for my marketing buck.*

In higher end referrals, your presence and your caregiver skill and LOOK must be high end (again, see Staffing).

The Bottom Line: Wherever your agency is located,

you are in the RIGHT territory with the WRONG mindset, skill or technique. Call your coach and get ideas. *Do not leave your territory until you receive referrals.*

✔ **"I can market two days a week, or three hours a day, or FROM HOME!"** I put trackers on my phones at one point, and many marketers try this one. Marketing is a self-directed, outside, field position, so if you are unorganized, low energy, lazy, or don't see results, you will eventually try Couch Marketing: calling people, "setting appointments," emailing, texting, messaging on social media—*anything but actually GOING to referral sources.*

Now, I have trust issues; and I believe that, once a marketer is not where they say they are, or does personal stuff during marketing hours, or lies, they either need a new position (in another company, preferably)—a position where they can be held accountable—or they need to begin being tracked by whether or not they actually get referrals. That is how I deal with outside staff.

The reason I know the tricks is because, after about two years of marketing myself, I began to do these same things—going home early, SAYING I was out marketing and really staying home. Hitting, like, two places then going shopping. Taking hundreds of Halloween promos to my friends and my kids instead of referral sources.

So if I can't stay motivated, how do my Franchise Partners or Marketers do it?

"Now, 18 years later, if I focus and spend two weeks somewhere, I am sure to get a referral. Why? Because I don't deviate from my focus. Every territory has referrals, no matter what they say."

When I see a lack of enthusiasm, I either recommend they *co-market* with a referral source (you know, one of those "friends" they have cultivated), go to a networking group, or I actually cut them back in hours and days. And for myself, I do the same. I say, "Okay, I will focus completely for three days until I see results." You cannot make money sitting at home, shopping, or anything else—and you are cheating yourself. If you suspect one of your marketers of doing it, they are cheating you. This is a boots on the ground business.

✔ **"I can keep my job and be successful."** At ABS we are finding more and more: *A mind divided is a dollar lost.* We have tried and tried this method, and as badly as we want our franchise partners to succeed—*they always fail when they try to begin this business alone and keep their previous employment.*

We are selling a future. We are investing in you being a successful Home Care Owner. You have already placed thousands of dollars on the table, and we are responsible for that, and for you.

We can no longer in good conscience take your money and allow you to become stressed, fearful, and overwhelmed while trying to work hard at, basically, what becomes two separate and opposing career paths, and then blame our product, or us—or have you blame yourself—because we are more vested in your success than even you are aware of, *and there is no way you can grow a business while working to make someone else rich.*

"This is a boots on the ground business."

You and your future deserve 100% of your time, energy and attention. Give us a year. You can always get another job! Your franchise investment may be just a drop in the bucket for you, but to us it means the difference between you having control of your future, building a meaningful legacy and becoming financially independent, versus doing the same things every day for someone else. So, no. You cannot keep your current employment and start a successful business, no matter what it is!

✔ **Getting overly familiar with your referral sources.** This is the *I am dropping the "Professional" stuff and "getting personal."* Not within the first six months you aren't! Even if your referral source has a weak moment and goes on a crying jag the second time you meet her, or gossips with you about someone else, or tells you something personal, make no mistake: You are still the Telemarketer on Legs, and it was a momentary lapse on their part.

Do NOT start off your next conversation with gossip, or by getting comfortable. As a marketer, you need to perfect the art of LISTENING more than talking (see Phase Two). I used to train marketers, and when we walked into a referral they would see me hug a referral source and so they would go in for a hug, too! Eek!

That hug took me YEARS to acquire. People do not like their personal space invaded by people they don't know. They do not like someone saying, "Hey, there!" the first or fifth time they meet. **They hold all of the cards and need — and WANT — to be treated as such.**

Do not get overly familiar. Stay calm and respectful, unless you see them out in the community. Even then, they may not recognize you. We are bothering them at work, so we need to remain aware of that, and not act like we are friends. We are not.

3. Phase One — The Basics: Preparing the Foundation for a Successful Entry into Marketing

✔ **Prepare a "Clean List."** When we set up your Territory, we will research your area and your listed referral sources on our mapping software. We will also, in your training, research other listed referral sources in your area.

A *Clean List,* however, is created by you once you have gone out, picked up business cards and listed your referral sources in your software system, with correct addresses, emails and contact names.

~Your first step to marketing success is to build a clean list in every city of your territory. Until you find EVERY hospital, skilled nursing facility, rehabilitation, therapist, home health agency, and hospice agency within that territory you are not done. You want to be detailed and specific on your list, with correct addresses and emails for contacts.

✔ **Generate your "Notes."** You will want to generate *Notes* regarding your referral sources to help you to remember what they say and when they are most available; who likes cookies and who likes healthy snacks.

~Keep a pad of paper with you, and collect business cards.

~Hit 5-10 places a day, then go home (or to the office) and prepare your notes and place them in your database while things are still fresh.

✔ **Maintain a "Marketing Log."** Your *Marketing Log* is a clean sheet of who you actually met, and who was unavailable. Place stars by places you think are better for you — "receptive," "friendly" — or where you know they utilize home care.

> *" Your first step to marketing success is to build a clean list in every city of your territory. Until you find EVERY hospital, skilled nursing facility, rehabilitation, therapist, home health agency, and hospice agency within that territory you are not done."*

✔ **Feel good about yourself.** Most professional marketers are a little arrogant, or at the very least, self-assured. As the owner, we have so many other things and worries on our mind that it can translate to insecurity, desperation, or fear, and that can manifest in many ways — not looking people in the eye, skipping places because we receive a less than warm welcome, talking too fast, nervously explaining our services, apologizing for disturbing the receptionist, trying too hard to please, and sometimes even being too pushy or downright rude because we think we are being brushed off.

Pro Tip: The best way to offset this heaviness and "feel good about yourself" is to set specific days you will market.

~Three days a week is the *least* our Franchise Partners can tolerate for success, and wake up with a plan!

~Have your list ready, or map out the new places for your list.

~Make yourself stay out at LEAST five hours, hitting as many spots as possible.

~Be friendly. Smile.

~In your first phase of marketing, you are just gathering information, so it is truly no big deal. So pep up and feel good about the progress you make each day!

~Be clean and neat. Wear business attire. You don't need a tie, although a nice button up shirt is preferred. Khakis or slacks for men, and a skirt or dress, or dress slacks, for women. Be presentable, and check yourself in the mirror before getting out of the car. *How you present yourself matters.*

Remember: You only get one chance to make a First Impression!

✔ **Bring just a few brochures/business cards.** Most professional marketers know this, but novices don't. They immediately ply the receptionist with cookies and gifts and they waste money very quickly.

~Your **first through third intro visits** are truly the fact finding phase—gathering information regarding the places you visit, taking tours in assisted livings, speaking with home health directors about the areas of service they perform, and becoming knowledgeable about THEM. Until you actually meet the person in charge, the pens, notepads, gummi bears and donuts need to wait. *You are feeding the receptionist, while she throws your brochures in the trash.*

~Leave ***two*** brochures and ***one*** business card until you get a chance to find out who does the referring. It feels bothersome, and many Franchisees say, "I feel stupid going in over and over. What do I say?"

~Until you meet with the Marketing person, Executive Director, Client Services Director, or Social Services Person, you continue to ask if you can set up a meeting, or you continue to leave your card and two brochures.

✔ **On the third visit you can bring "Trinkets and Trash"**—cookies, candy bar, note pad, pens, *with the understanding that the actual referral source may never see them, but the receptionist will begin to love you.*

"Until you actually meet the person in charge, the pens, notepads, gummi bears and donuts need to go. You are feeding the receptionist, while she throws your brochures in the trash."

✔ **Get to know your Referral Sources.** Until you know what THEY do, how do you expect them to care what YOU do? Competition is fierce. And in business, as in life, we like people who ask questions about us, who are genuinely interested in what we do and who we are, people who smile and enjoy their time with us, and definitely people who RETAIN some knowledge of what and who we are. The same goes for business.

Pro Tip: Use *their* terminology for their business. I used to make the same mistake over and over, calling Assisted Livings a "Facility," when they refer to themselves as a "Community." It's a seemingly small mistake, but over and over I showed the referral source that I was NOT LISTENING when we spoke, and as a result I had to work twice as hard for referrals.

It's nice to be able to ask in the correct place, "What is your Census?" "How many beds do you have?" "Do you accept Medicare or Medi-Cal, Access, or Medicaid?"

When you know the receptionist by name and the person in charge by *title and name,* you are ready to go into Phase Two.

4. Phase Two—Marketing 101: Beginning The Process of Building Successful Relationships

Lia's Story:
A Successful Relationship Will Carry You Far

An example of this is a great DSD (Director of Staff Development) who I created a relationship with while doing her registry. Not only did she give me over $60K worth of registry business for her skilled nursing facility, but, when she left that facility and moved to another, she kicked out their registry and brought me in there – to the tune of about $40K a month. I genuinely like her; and because I do good business and stay on top of her staffing, she likes me, too. As a result, I have been given over $100K worth of business from ONE PERSON. Now that is a successful business relationship!

~~~

30 Days In

✔ **Become the "Known Face."** At this point, you have been to the facility/community three to four times and your first 30 days are over. Now you will begin plying them with LITTLE treats. (By little, I mean *cheap*!) I am partial to Wal-Mart cookies ($2.99 per pack), Wal-Mart candy bars (you can get the 6-pack of snack bars for one dollar), note pads/sticky pads or pens (one or two—not a lot).

Pro Tip: EVERY OTHER time you go, bring something. Not "every" time. And don't hang out when you do—these are drop offs! You now know who to ask for, and you have created a **small** relationship with the receptionist (always leave her something on these treats stops, too). *So now you can say, "Hey Lisa, can you take these to Sarah? Thank you!"*

✔ **Begin your Placement Contract gathering and marketing.** (See Chapter 7 on Placement.) This allows you to begin with a free service request and gets your name out there as a Potential Assisted Living Community Partner—and a helpful facility referral source.

You have something to ask that is NOT about home care, and *they love NOT being sold.* This is how you begin to develop a good relationship. *This works amazingly at hospitals.*

60 to 90 Days In

✔ **Begin ASKING for the business.** This could be a whole chapter by itself, because it is crucial to your success to learn and perfect "asking for business"—the right way.

~At this point, you have been in the facility, community, rehabilitation, assisted living, etc. for about 60 to 90 days—at least 21 visits—so take your time, and cultivate the **name-company recognition factor**.

~When you walk in, they may say, "I just gave out your brochure!"—the quintessential lie every referral source says to continue getting your candy and other goods, and so they don't feel bad when you come in. But...you have received no calls?

"I have moved into first position many times by being Johnny On The Spot second choice."

You have received no requests for service from ANY clients that have been in this facility—so now comes the balancing act between calling their bluff and remaining respectful.

An appropriate response would be, "Have you had any discharges home?" And if they have already said that they gave out your brochure, the question is—not aggressively, "What is the name, so I can keep an eye out for them?"

They may get cagey at this point, and say, "I don't recall," or, "They didn't need it," or some other excuse. Then you can respond with, "Okay, thank you so much for thinking about me. Is there anyone going home this week that I can talk to while I am here?"

This only works at Skilled Nursing facilities, Hospitals and Rehabilitation Centers—all of your others, AL/IL, etc.—are not sending people home. So the question would be, "Are there any residents that have been taken to the hospital I can visit?"

Now comes the moment of truth: Do they TRULY want to refer to you when they say, "No," or, "Let me check on that"?

Pro Tip: A good idea is to offer a free service: "If I speak with anyone directly at your facility, I will give them the first 4 hours free so they can try me out." And then *gently* exit stage left. Come back with candy or treats in two or three days, chat up the receptionist and ask her, "Anyone going home?" or, "Anyone in the hospital?"

Until it feels comfortable, variations of this can include, "Is anyone needing to be discharged to a community or facility?" Remember, you have placement contracts, so you can also help with that.

~Your new intro after **90 days** should be, "Great to see you — I have some great caregivers available, is anyone going home today or this week?"

> *"How you handle your first case will determine whether you receive the bulk of the business or remain always in second or third position."*

And then it becomes easy and natural.

Pro Tip: You can offer transportation. You should have been listening to their needs and spoken to your ABS coach about the things they may need so you can begin tailoring your conversations to *helping* them rather than taking *from* them.

✔ **Little mind tricks to stay motivated.** Okay, so you are feeling like a stalker, and perhaps they roll their eyes when you come in. I commonly hear, "But it's been 45 days and they aren't giving me business. I feel like I have nothing left to say. I feel stupid."

Start asking yourself: "How many people do I know in the facility/hospital/referral source?" If the answer is, "Um, the receptionist and the SW," then that is too few.

~Start bringing candy to other areas of your referral source, start saying hello to everyone in the place! *See how many people you can get to know over the next 30 days.* I start in elevators—saying hello and how are you doing to any and all staff members I see. I will go to nursing stations and leave pens and sticky pads or notes at the station.

~I like to figure out how long people have been with the company and what they do. I like to find out if there is anything "free" that I can offer that won't break the bank but allows me a little grace—like the aforementioned "free transportation." Or a free two hour shower visit?

~Another thing to remember is you are only bringing in a few brochures at a time, giving rate sheets, and maybe even creating newsletters and information sheets to drop off. Do you know who does their marketing? Are you on a first name basis?

~If it is an Assisted Living, have you referred anyone yet? Do you have their information? Can you talk about that?

✔ **Next game is, "Who Are They Referring Business To?"** This takes some digging, but that is the second question (once you are in the community and they are really comfortable with you and you know more people).

You HAVE to know WHY you aren't getting the business — and a lot of the time it boils down to the fact that they already have a relationship with another agency. If you know WHO, you can begin to find out what that agency DOESN'T provide: Is it transportation? Is it short shifts? What do they charge?

~Research the other agency, maybe even marketing them for any cases or small shifts they don't want.

~Then begin again *intelligently* asking for the business: "I know you guys use Company X, but if you want two hours only, I can do that," or transportations, or, "I'd like to be your second choice."

I have moved into first position many times by being Johnny On The Spot. We all make mistakes, and the problem is, once we land an account (see Phase Three, below), we all tend to get lazy. *And so will the facility's current first choice.*

~When they slip, you will get a frantic call (only if you have followed Phases One and Two; if not, someone else will get the call) and you will get the opportunity to show them what you are made of, which usually involves calling every caregiver on your roster and begging them to go to work NOW and do a great job!

Bottom Line: This is where, if you have a second job, or when you are unfocused...*or if you haven't interviewed and hired enough caregivers*...you will lose your opportunity.

If you have a second job, the call comes in, you are AT WORK, and you can't help them. If you stopped hiring caregivers because you felt bad about not having work—now you have called all six of your caregivers and they are all working, not answering, or can't go until tomorrow. (Just imagine your odds if you had hired 25!)

Now you are ready for Phase 3.

5. Phase 3—Going Deep, Not Wide: Relationship Strategies For Ongoing Progress

✔ **"Thank you and goodbye." What NOT To Do.** So the referral source gives you your first case! Yaaay! You are excited, you staff it, and then you sit and wait for another one. You may say, "Thank you!" And then you are on to the next referral source. (Hence, "Thank you and goodbye.")

But, where there is one case there are others. So when you get that first case—even if it is only one hour—that is where you begin your *real* relationship building. How you handle your first case will determine whether you receive the bulk of the business or remain always in second or third position.

"Like friendships we neglect, which tend to fall away—referral sources are no exception. Right behind you is another company with a fresh faced marketer who understands the concept better than you do."

✔ **What TO Do.** Whenever you get a new case, ask

who referred your agency, and:

~*Immediately* put a Thank You card in the mail, to both the referral source and to the potential client. (You can find these in the ABS Portal.)

~Once the client is on service, call your referral and leave a voice mail regarding when it starts and who is staffed.

~When the case has had a few days of service, *go to the client's home, and check on things.* If they are extremely happy, ask them to call the person who recommended you and let them know the caregiver gets a kudos, if they do.

~On your next visit to the referral source, bring something better than usual: a dozen donuts, cookies—something the referral source can share, AND something especially for them (small, like a coffee gift card), and let them know how the case is going. Mention that you have gone by and visited.

~Continue to visit that referral source *twice a week.* Don't always ask for them, but keep dropping off little things until you are receiving more referrals, so they know you were there—without disturbing them too much.

~Then, drop back to *once a week*, always checking in.

✔ **"I haven't heard from you in a while."** This is usually because you have disappeared and not gone by. (Again…"Thank you, and goodbye.")

The biggest problem with most marketers is:
The grass is always greener on the other side (or at
the other place). The grass is actually just fine where
you are getting referrals from.

Pro Tip: Do not cultivate more referral sources than you can focus on. Like friendships we neglect, which tend to fall away—referral sources are no exception. Right behind you is another company with a fresh faced marketer who understands the concept better than you do.

"(W)hen you get that first case—even if it is
only one hour—that is where you begin your
real relationship building."

"I haven't heard from you in a while." This statement is a RED FLAG when a referral source uses it, or, "I've missed seeing you lately." Those things translate to, "I am giving your cases to someone else."

Now, they won't say that. What they WILL say is, "I just gave out your brochure." But, truly? They are letting you know subtly that you aren't doing your job.

✔ **I personally like to focus on ONE area, two times a week.** Why?

~It is easier on gas.

~I don't have to meet new people.

~I can go to the same places over and over.

~I can become the recognizable face.

~BECAUSE IT WORKS.

✔ **"They Never Refer." When To Move On, Or When To Hire Someone Else**. My motto and feeling on this is, there are NO BAD referral sources.

The most common statement I hear is: "They don't refer to anyone," or, "You can never get in there." Well, my answer is always, *Someone is getting the referrals—it is just not YOU.* Or, perhaps you are pitching the wrong service line.

Eventually, in these cases, move on until you have a team. Then you can switch up to find out who works best at that location.

> *"How you handle your first case will determine whether you receive the bulk of the business or remain always in second or third position."*

Until then, a rule of thumb is: If, after 90 days of hitting a referral source 2-3 times a week, you are not even getting a Transportation, and if you have only seen the receptionist for those 90 days, *then you have failed to connect to the right person.*

✔ **On the Verge.** So you are in one territory with 25 places on your list. You hit all 25 twice a week, with cookies, small things ("Trinkets and Trash"), and you are becoming well known. After two months you have received referrals from three of the 25 places.

Okay, now you can move to the next territory — but you must incorporate those three places into your route. So you move to the next 25 referral sources, and you hit those AND the three you have received referrals from — TWICE a week.

Bottom Line: You only need referrals from 10 places to grow, but you need ALL of the referrals from those ten places.

So you will continue with:

~60 to 90 days in the same small area, adding those who refer to you into your rotation, and…

~Create a list based off of WHO ACTUALLY REFERS. Note who is on your list. This should be documented in your database software system.

Pro Tip: Until you have a Marketing Team that you can teach this method to, *your whole goal is to develop only 10-15 Great Referral Sources, and then leave the rest alone.*

It will minimize your workload. It will make your relationships stronger, more focused. Your referral sources will know that you are consistent and trustworthy, and it allows you to do good business.

The problem is, when you go WIDE, you become sporadic at best and people are giving you two hour shifts instead of 12 hour shifts. Why? Because you are not the Preferred Provider.

"If, after 90 days of hitting a referral source 2-3 times a week you are not even getting a Transportation, but if you have only seen the receptionist for those 90 days, you will be actually leaving before you have even begun."

6. Highest Marketing Status: PREFERRED PROVIDER

This is where you want to be with 5-10 of your referral sources.

A "Preferred Provider" or "Preferred Vendor" is just what it says—that you are THE vendor or caregiving provider within the facility, hospital, or nursing home.

Lia's Story:
What Being a Preferred Provider Can Do For You

I had a referral source who would say, "I only use Lia" — not A Better Solution — but Lia. Once a month I took her to lunch, and weekly I STILL brought her staff donuts, cookies and such. She was referring two great cases a WEEK. And: She was creating a barrier to other agencies trying to get into her facility. She was the Admissions person.

How long did this take? Three YEARS! Why? Because I didn't have this book to help me, and I would hit her for a month and then disappear and assume she had no referrals to give.

When I finally realized that she actually LIKED me, and I got tired of marketing everywhere else, and she was right down the street from my office — I finally became consistent, and after three months I was Preferred. That lasted for four years, until they hired a discharge planner. To this day, if SHE can, she will refer to me; but most of the referrals aren't hers.

I kept going, however, probably once a week, and her Administrator gave me my first "Supplemental Staffing" referral, and it has become a huge part of my business.

~~~

Bottom Line: Becoming "Preferred" is no easy feat. There is competition out there, and people go places every other day. But usually they are different places. So pick 25 and stay in them for 90 days and go twice a week. Be consistent, and you will achieve preferred vendor status and be the only referral for certain places.

Understand that Preferred Status makes you almost a "Friend" to your referral source, so be prepared to do things every few months outside of work, if that allows—a Happy Hour, lunch or even just checking in without ever talking about business.

Maintaining that relationship is very difficult — they also must be one of your vendors, so you have to dig in and…

✔ **Find out what they need**. One of my first preferred provider accomplishments was with an admissions social worker at a Skilled Nursing Facility (or

Convalescent, Post-Acute, referred to as a SNF). What she needed to know was, "How are the OTHER skilled places doing?" So when I was out marketing, I would see who had open beds, and I would let her know what her competition looked like.

Always keep in mind:

~What do they need?

~How can you provide it?

~How can you enrich *their* job, position, community awareness?

~Do you place *their* brochures in *your* packets?

~Do you place people in *their* facility?

~Do you bring goodies for their whole staff monthly or so?

"There is competition out there, and people go places every other day. But usually they are different places, so pick 25 and stay in them for 90 days and go twice a week."

~Do you still watch over their cases or initial referrals and give feedback? Even after six months? Two years? Most marketers don't. This is where they say, "Thank you, goodbye," and, "My Field Supervisor has it," or they take their eye off of the cases.

They begin to take the Referral for granted.

Pro Tip: Mediocre Marketers by their very nature are selfish, a tad lazy, and not detail-oriented. They want their cake and eat it, too.

So remember: If a marketer has Preferred Status, you, as the owner, need to show *your* face and say thank you. Because your Marketer, Field Supervisor, whomever, will drop the ball eventually, and you need to be able to pick up the pieces after they have forgotten the work it took for them to receive the referrals.

7. Marketing Tip: Partnering Up

This is one of my favorite ways of combating the boredom and constant repetition of showing up at the same places every day — with the same thing to sell. I "Bring a Friend." It is very helpful, because I can then introduce someone new into the mix.

By now, you have met with the Executive Director, Administrator, Case Manager, etc., and they have maybe referred, maybe not — do they have a Marketer?

✔ **Everyone has a Bottom Line.** EVERYONE in this industry wants the same thing — Patients, Clients, Residents — SOMEONE to buy what they are selling. Just because your referral source is not the one "selling," it doesn't mean that they are unconcerned with their bottom line, and they would love for you to help them with that.

✔ **The question is: "Do you want to market with me?"**

This can only happen when you have established a marketing route and actually are marketing to people who might help your referral source grow. If this is a Skilled Nursing or Assisted Living in one town and you only market three towns over to other Assisted Livings, then that is not helpful. If no one knows you? You guessed it: That is not helpful.

✔ **Develop a route based on your referral source's needs** and take their Marketing person, their receptionist, etc., with you. Sometimes they have valuable referral sources for you as well, but don't butt in or cut them off. Subtly introduce them. *This is you being courteous.* You are almost marketing FOR them.

Bottom Line: Do this monthly. It keeps you from getting bored and allows the community to see who you partner with, giving you more credibility.

✔ **Remember to never market with anyone who does the exact same thing as you do** — unless you both have your niche and they either are *larger* than you or they have *more referrals* than you.

✔ **Please leave your BAD habits and "loose" conversation at home**. Do NOT talk about too many personal issues. Do not talk about how you "usually go home at 2." Do not talk about flaws or mess ups within your company. Sensing the trend here? Try to do more LISTENING than talking.

✔ **Talk about the referrals you get and how you convert, or how they convert**. Find out about the company structure. WATCH. Observe.

Learning how *they* market can teach you tips and help you to be a better marketer.

CHAPTER 7
PLACEMENT

(What is Placement?)

Placement is the business of placing people who are discharging from a hospital or facility — or who cannot remain at home — into a community or assisted living or a board and care facility that works within their budget, location and specific care needs, whereby you get a percentage of their first month's rent in that community or facility.

Selling placements is your beginning sales point.

Lia's Story:
Lessons Learned, Placement Lost

I once had a 24-hour, around the clock, client that we had been servicing for over two years suddenly alert my staffer (who informed me) that she would be going into a facility the following week, so service was ending. That was a big chunk of change to lose, but I understood.

What I didn't understand was why my Field Supervisor, or

Care Manager, didn't know ahead of time that our client was looking for a community. And that our client's family didn't know we do placement! We lost revenue AND the capability to provide ALL of the services we could have — because we didn't sell completely.

~~~

1. What is Needed?

✔ **Contracts.** The first thing that you have to establish is contracts within the assisted living and facility community. A Better Solution Franchise system provides you with those. We personally contract for 80% of the first month's rent. This is a great time to market, because you are *not asking for anything* — you are *giving* through the opportunity to assist in filling up a community or board and care.

✔ First, tour the facility and get to know the administrator, marketing person, receptionist, and all of the other management staff.

2. What You Are Looking For

✔ **Price point.** What is the price point? You need to have a range of different price options available for your placements. Find the lowest option up to the highest. Remember to ask a few things:

~Is this the **Base Rate** or an **All Inclusive Rate**? There is a large range. They may advertise $2,750 per month, but by the time they are done with Add-Ons, it could be as high as $6,000.

~What are the additions? Most communities or assisted livings have tiers or levels, and they go up quickly in price for little things, so you want to know ALL of the hidden fees.

✔ **Who does the assessments and what are the requirements?** Depending on your state, the usual requirement is a physician's report. You should have those on hand so you can facilitate that yourself and expedite placement.

Get to know the expectation of the person doing the assessment—some will bend the rules and take difficult residents, some will not. And *this person is a great referral source for you,* as they can recommend home care when someone isn't suitable for their community.

✔ **How is the food?** Have lunch there. As we get older, food is one of the few pleasures we have left, and we need to know the quality of the food being served and the choices, so make sure you have lunch there. *This knowledge will come in handy, as will the incidental networking you do while there.*

✔ **What do the rooms look like?**

✔ **Resident Relations:** How does the staff treat and care for the residents?

✔ **Ratio:** What is the ratio of caregiver to client? Learn the industry standard for ratios in Assisted Living and Memory Care in your area.

✔ **Skilled Professionals On-Site?** Do they have a Memory Care? Do they have a Skilled unit? They call these anything from Healthcare Centers ("Vanguard") to Skilled Nursing Facilities, but the most expensive communities have one on campus so Residents don't have to leave the campus as their health declines.

3. What is Optimum?

✔ **Having at least 25-30 contracts in three different areas of town** — ranging from the rock bottom ($900 per month board and care) to the very top ($6,500-$7,500 assisted living or facility).

✔ **Having relationships within that facility or community** — and knowing what specials they are running, and what types of rooms they have available.

✔ **Being knowledgeable.** You must be able to tell family members as much as they need to know about each facility before they tour.

4. How Do I Get Placements?

✔ **Find your minimum placement option.** Hospitals and skilled nursing are always discharging patients who cannot go home without care and who cannot afford the amount of care they need.

Many times they will attempt to give you placements on Social Security or with very limited funding ability.

If you do not have any facilities, board and care, or

communities under $1,200 then find a placement agency who does. *Do NOT say no — but do not waste too much time on Non-Paying Placement.*

Pro Tip: If you do not have a contract — get one in place before the Patient/Client or their family even visits.

✔ **When you assess home care clients, make sure they KNOW you do placements.** Many times they will have home care but are looking for placements, and they are using someone else, because it hasn't been made clear.

✔ **Involve the client's family in the Placement "pitch."** Placement is a *family* decision to move someone out of their home. Remember, in many cases you are selling to the children or spouse more than to the client.

✔ **Meet them at the community or facility.** That way you can better assess their situation and answer any questions, and so they can feel comfortable.

Remember:
Selling Placements is Your Beginning Sales Point.

Bottom Line: Placement is a FREE service to the client, and it helps the skilled nursing move lower end custodial patients to make room for higher paying "Skilled Need" patients.

✔ **Selling Placements is the easiest way to create, and open doors for, relationships.** It allows you to create a database of communities and facilities that know who you are and who can go to you with questions, or service needs, once you begin placing in communities and facilities. *It will be easier to ASK them for the home care business and build a Transitional Package for them.*

✔ **Continually remind clients and their families that it is part of your service line.**

✔ **Selling them yourself versus partnering with Placement Agencies:** There are plenty of "Placement Only" agencies to partner with if you do not have enough personnel or time to perform the task of getting contracts and walking the family through the process. Remember, though, that most smaller placement agencies charge YOU to refer Home Care, *so beware of the trap.* Make sure you partner with a placement agency that doesn't charge.

I highly recommend you develop this service line on your own.

CHAPTER 8
INTAKE

(What is Intake?)

First things first: An *Intake* is an inquiry; an exchange of information between you (or your staff) and a potential client that is captured in writing, discussed, and—if you are lucky—it is "closed" on the phone, but not often.

At this stage in the game, if you have worked really hard and applied all of the lessons above, then— *viola!*—you have gotten that call! And you are so excited that your hands are shaking and you practically barrel over the person on the other end of the phone with all of the wonderful things you can do for them; or even WORSE, you haven't said *anything*, just stammered and chit chatted...and they say they will call you back...or they are checking around and "will let you know," or you have just picked up the message from your cell phone—an hour or two after the call—and are now stalking the caller like a rejected ex-lover. This is the most important call you will ever receive as a Home Care owner! So everything stops with this call.

When I started my company, I had only myself and a friend helping me four hours a day answering phones and hiring caregivers. My business cards had the office number, and when she got a call, she would take down the vital information and call me. I have pulled over on the freeway, stopped marketing, ended conversations abruptly—whatever I was doing halted when she made that call. And cell phones were barely out then.

I could have called while driving; it wasn't illegal yet! But I needed to *write* the information down. It is and will always be your FIRST interaction with the actual sales process, and you need to understand the importance of it.

"This is the most important call you will ever receive as a Home Care owner! So everything stops with this call."

This is your money. This is your opportunity to provide someone with excellent care. To prove to your referral source you are the best agency. To provide a person with a job that may feed their family.

This Intake is *everything* to you!

1. How To Make That Intake Call Count:

✔ **Stop whatever you are doing, and have a pen and paper ready (preferably an intake form).**

✔ **Speak slowly and clearly. And Listen.**

✔ **The Vital Information — Asking the 5 W's:**

~Who are they? (Potential client? Family member? Neighbor?) And how can you contact them?

~What hours are they thinking of having care?

~Where did they hear about you?

~When do they want service to start?

~Why are they needing care?

2. Developing on the 5 W's: Build slowly on these during the call.

✔ **Who?** Usually the call is made by a family member; sometimes by the client themselves. Needing care is a very stressful thing, so *who they are* is more than just information — it is a conversation you need to have once you have gathered the information.

~*Start with & always get:* Name, Phone Number, Email, Street Address or Area of Town — FIRST.

Bottom Line: You need to relax and listen. Do not rush someone. If you are too busy for an intake, you are too busy to own a Home Care Agency. This is a service where we help people in NEED, and they need your attention and your understanding, and — ultimately — your expertise on how you can help.

✔ **What Hours?** This is not set in stone until you meet

them, and they often overestimate their own ability to care for themselves, so do not be discouraged by the person who says, "I want ONE hour." Go see them. They may not be able to walk—they may have fallen or be confused. *They may need more assistance and just not understand it.*

✔ **Where did they hear about you?** This is a MUST. Find out who you need thank and report to about this client. Sometimes they won't remember, but during the in-person assessment, find out where they are coming from, if they received a brochure, who else is involved—Hospice? Home Health?—and that way you can get a general idea of how to best provide service.

"If you are too busy for an intake, you are too busy to own a Home Care Agency. This is a service where we help people in NEED, and they need your attention and your understanding."

✔ **When?** This is crucial. Some people want it NOW. I like those calls, but many do not. They become frantic and start thinking, "What if I can't?" "Who do I have?"

Well, from my perspective, "now" usually means a two hour window *and I can usually go start it myself.*

What "now" really means is that, if I say YES...

~I get the case—no more calling around, no beating out another agency: I don't have to wait—it's in the bag!

~I can charge what I want, no haggling: They need care *now*. I don't gouge if it is 6 hours or more. But if it is 2-4 hours, I charge very high ($3 or $4 dollars above my minimum) because it is harder to staff, and I pay top dollar for short shifts.

~But even if "When" is next month—get over there IMMEDIATELY. It is not your case until the contract is signed! So go meet with them quickly.

✔ **Why?** The diagnosis. Critical info! Are they walking? Needing a full lift transfer? Violent? Broken hip? Bed bound? You need to know for pricing and staffing what is wrong with your client, so ask a LOT of questions.

Our intake form has many questions and the care plan we complete in person has even more. The more I know about my clients' needs the better I can match them up. (See Chapter 9—Staffing.)

3. Set a Range.

You have done your homework. You have been in the field, you know what other agencies in your state, city, county are charging. Now you give a range. In San Diego, California we are currently at $23-$28 per hour. Arizona may be $19-$22 per hour. Kansas may be $18-$20 per hour. Know the range for your city and set your margins. (See Chapter 12 on Margins.) You will then be able to *sell your value*.

4. Set a time—the sooner the better—to get that Assessment.

This is your whole end game: Getting in front of the person who needs care, or their family. This is also your "Interview" of them—and they of you. You are often up against other agencies, based on referral source recommendation.

"It is not your case until the contract is signed!"

5. The Assessment

✔ **Be ON TIME.**

✔ **Be Neat and Presentable.**

✔ **If you have time, speak with the referral source first.** Find out what they recommend for this client, so you can mention that.

✔ **Acknowledge the client directly.** Even if they are in a hospital bed—Say "Hello." *Show care and concern.*

✔ **Find out the expectations** that the family or client will have for your caregiver.

✔ **Offer your services to contact the discharge planner**, or referral source, to set up care.

✔ **Remind them that the more lead time you have to choose a caregiver the better the fit will be.** That, if they call you right before discharge, they will get whoever is available for their hours, but if they give you 2-3 days leeway you have time to interview and explain the needs to prospective caregivers.

✔ **Offer free training** if there is time before start of care. (Two hours MAX.)

✔ **Offer a reassessment of needs** after one week.

✔ **Talk to them about what they need** — there is always a discrepancy between what THEY think they need and what you KNOW they need. So *gently* work them to a higher number of hours to start with and then a reassessment to lower. This is based on safety and to ensure proper staffing.

"Selling is listening."

Your caregiver won't want to leave a fragile person alone after three or four hours, so if there is no support at home, we recommend more hours at first and gradually lowering service hours as they rehabilitate.

6. Closing the Deal — What TO Do

✔ **Leave them with your folder and a filled out service agreement.** No one in the process likes to make a decision right away, so pressing them to sign can be a turn off. Instead encourage them to look it over, and explain that it is not "time-binding," but rather *rate and service expectation*, and a *procedural* agreement, between the both of you.

Read your Service Agreement and commit it to memory.

Also explain, fully, how you bill, and that *service CANNOT begin without a signed agreement.* Make sure you have address and email information. And that they have your business card and cell phone number for more questions.

7. The Follow Up

Pro Tip: When you finish, immediately send out a "Thank you for your time" card, with your business card inside. That will help you stand out from the competition.

✔ **Sell VALUE not PRICE**. I personally interview all of my own caregivers (or my caregivers go through a rigorous interview process). Explain what you are doing to ensure Quality of Care, and what makes you different. Do you do weekly phone calls? Do your caregivers have Medical Insurance? Do you have Care Management visits? Do the clients have YOUR personal cell phone number?

What do you do to make your Price Point worth their choice?

✔ **More follow up:** Go in and speak with your referral source again and let them know your observations, rates and what you have offered. Thank them, and the next day bring in donuts for them.

✔ **Visit the client regularly if they are not discharging soon.**

✔ **Prepping the talent:** Speak to a few caregivers who

fit the need and check their availability.

✔ **Call the family after 24 hours.** See if they have made a decision, and let them know you have one or two caregivers for them to meet if they would like.

8. Closing the Deal — What NOT to Do

✔ **Do not promise the moon** — and either *not* deliver, or cut the price. If you cut the price, you are not making margins.

✔ **Do not set up interviews more than a week before care will start**. Caregivers will be unavailable. (See Chapter 9 — Staffing.)

So what do you do to make your Price Point worth their choice?

✔ **Again — Do not make promises you cannot keep.**

✔ **Do not rush for a sales pitch** — *selling is listening.*

✔ **Do not assume you have the case.**

✔ **Do not forget to follow up.**

✔ **Do not create an unprofessional environment** — by getting overly familiar, or talking about personal stuff too much.

✔ **Do not forget to ask everyone in the family's opinion** — and be interested.

✔ **Do not let them drive the care:** Be the expert.

Bottom Line: Whether they choose your agency or not, you want them to be better off because they met you.

CHAPTER 9
STAFFING

1. Phase One — Finding That Match

You got the case! This is when the real work starts. Up until now the focus has been on you, the network of professionals, the families and the clients. Now we go through another variable — and this one is the most important: Assigning the caregiver.

The hardest part in the beginning is actually finding one that is available for work at the specific hours that are needed, to start on the DAY the client would like...and who is available to meet the client prior, likes the client, wants to work... Just add a hodge podge of other "issues" to your mix of home care staffing challenges and you'll see why I say that this is the hardest part — in the beginning. Follow these guidelines, however, and you'll find staffing to run fairly smoothly.

✔ **Make sure you have the hours SET.** Caregivers have lives, and you wouldn't want someone calling you and saying, "Hey, *maybe* can you work tomorrow? Ummm, two, six, or possibly 12 hours?" But that is what we do, and then we claim the CAREGIVERS are flaky!

✔ **Make a decision and sell the TRUTH**. Caregivers need work to feed their families, so the more hours, the more likely they are to have fewer changes.

✔ **Establish the parameters of the case.**

~Set the hours. First things first. As stated above, we cannot ask a caregiver to reserve time to work for "maybes." *Set hours mean fewer changes.*

~Set the days. Be honest and let the client and caregiver know up front what the case requires. Two-hour shifts will not get consistent caregivers, as they need full-time work, but you need to be able to promise to place skilled caregivers on "Visits" (the term for under four hours).

~If the hours are less than four, charge more—so you can PAY more. If you are paying $12 for 8 hours, pay $14 for 3 hours—*that will create an incentive for your caregivers to accept and remain on the case.*

~If the client wants a changing schedule (not "fixed"), then you should require a minimum number of hours, preferably 35, so they can have one caregiver who is available to them, ensuring that the caregiver can make enough money to not leave.

~*Do not let the client drive the care.* If the client is a fall risk and they only want an hour in the evening—who will be checking on them at night? Or early morning? Try to add the hours the client NEEDS—not the hours they THINK they need.

~All schedule changes come through the office. Make sure both caregiver and client know that they are responsible for the hours contracted, and shortening hours or schedule changes need to come through the office or they will result in billing errors—*or even caregiver termination*—if the caregiver isn't on an expected shift.

"Make sure you have the hours SET. Caregivers have lives, and you wouldn't want someone calling you and saying, 'Hey, "maybe" can you work tomorrow?'"

✔ **Put your best foot forward.** Make sure on your first 8-10 cases you place HIGHLY SKILLED and PRESENTABLE caregivers. Period.

~Pay your caregivers on the first 8-10 cases the highest rate.

~Create a "base" of exceptional workers. Set the bar high.

~If you have a roster of 15 caregivers that you hired at $11 per hour and you get chosen for your first case, offer the caregivers you like the most $13 per hour—and if they do well, and create a great reputation for you, KEEP paying them that.

~Having 3 or 4 that are your "go to" caregivers means that they are presentable and skilled, and clients really like them. Paying them better means that *the loss of your margins will be offset by the boost to your reputation.*

~Word of mouth is your largest referral source.

~Highly skilled means "Top Picks." (See below.)

✔ **Calling all Caregivers!** Our software system at A Better Solution allows us to send out a mass text to all of our caregivers at once. That is what I do first.

~The minute I get a case that has substantial hours, I send a text with "Case Open in Egypt. 35 hours per week—Please Call."

~Then I begin calling my top picks for the case.

~Call those that meet the criteria first, and then *answer the call* when those that receive the text start calling back.

Pro Tip: The best caregiver for the case is usually the LAST one to call back—so the best practice is to staff it with a caregiver who fits the bill, and when your TOP PICK calls in, replace the other caregiver with them.

~*Availability* doesn't mean someone who can work *half* of a 20-hour a week case. The best match is someone who can do *all* of the hours (40 or less in OT states) that are requested by the client.

✔ **Top Picks: Play your first string…first.**

Top Picks—you need to have at least five of these for every 25 caregivers on your roster:

~These are the caregivers that you think will do the best job for the case. They are usually the ones you *don't mind* paying a little more, too.

~They are the ones that always look the part, say the right thing and present well.

~They are the ones who are professional and kind.

"Word of mouth is your largest referral source."

~They are also the ones that you have good rapport with, who can roll with the punches.

~They are the ones that you can place two days on every case—*and every case wants them full time.*

~They are also the ones that you may have so spread out that you will lose them—if you're not careful. (See Phase Two below—Scheduling the Caregiver.)

✔ **Pulling players off the bench.** Second and Third String Caregivers are the ones you use when a TOP PICK is unavailable.

~They are presentable, but English may not be their first language—making them harder for older clients.

~They may not conduct themselves as well as you'd like.

~They may be inconsistent—one clients loves them, two clients have complaints.

~They may not look or present as "neat" consistently.

~They may not always be on time.

~They may be those that call off twice a month...EVERY month.

~They may have limited availability (Tuesdays and Thursdays between 3 and 8, etc.).

~They may be too talkative about personal issues.

> *"'Availability' doesn't mean someone who can work half of a 20-hour-a-week case. The best match is someone who can do all of the hours (40 or less in OT states) that are requested by the client."*

~They may not like certain office staff—and that may be you.

~They may have a limited skill set, not be able to lift, or handle certain clients.

~They may be reliable—but very picky.

✔ **Explain the case—completely & correctly.**

Bottom Line: Explain everything that, to you, seems really, really obvious.

~Give all of the correct information. Again, seems obvious, but you'd be surprised.

~Do not be cagey or manipulative when staffing. It is natural to worry about being turned down, but when we don't give accurate information, we place our caregivers in a bad situation or feeling underprepared, and at times they will walk off—or tell the client that they "did not know," or "were not informed," which makes your agency look very unprofessional.

~When you give information, if you can and while you are smaller, try to meet with the caregiver beforehand, and help them feel confident about the job they are going to perform and the person they are caring for.

~Never assume someone has received information when you have spoken with them directly: A lot of caregivers and nurses like to receive instructional texts or emails. That is fine as long as they confirm that they have received it.

 "Top Picks—you need to have at least five of these for every 25 caregivers on your roster."

~Communicate new information as you receive it—even minor client complaints or concerns—but *be respectful of your caregivers, as they are sensitive to criticism and they are working with your clients.*

~Look up directions yourself and place in client's file,

in your database. That way ANYONE can guide the caregiver to the client's home; or if a new caregiver is going, they have access and a better chance of being prepared.

✔ **Interviews between clients & caregivers.** Try not to set up interviews too far in advance — your caregivers are always looking for work, *and you must explain this to your clients.* They think picking a caregiver is like packing for a trip — the sooner you do it the more prepared you are. That is not true. The earlier you choose a caregiver, the LESS likely it will be that the caregiver will be available when you need her/him.

~Make sure you have a signed contract. Do not just push for the interview. Without a contract, the client is not committed.

~Do not send all of one nationality, personality, or body type. Give the clients a choice and always send out two caregivers for any case over 25 hours.

~Do not OFFER interviews. You have to pay your caregivers, and some clients will literally scare the caregivers off in the interviews, or they will become incredibly picky — "I want a college degree" type of thing. Or the perfect caregiver goes in and says, "No, I can't start at 7, only 8," and you are sitting there looking perplexed! *And you still have to pay every caregiver that interviews* depending on your state labor law.

2. Phase Two — Best Practices in Staffing and Caregiver Etiquette for Your "Brand Ambassadors" (a.k.a. Troubleshooting)

✔ **How to speak to (and treat) your Caregivers/Nurses.** Many people call Caregivers and Nurses a "Low Wage Work Force" and recommend you "understand" how to deal with or "manage" them. But the truth is, in this day and age, they are just like your six figure friends—living paycheck to paycheck. The difference is the education level, as well as the stress level of their careers.

~The stress level of the caregiver/nurse's job creates a tense atmosphere if communication isn't handled carefully.

~Caregivers are sensitive by nature, or they couldn't care for others.

~And on the flipside, caregivers know that, once the client likes them, they have the upper hand.

~Caregivers need clear and direct communication.

"The stress level of the caregiver/nurse's job creates a tense atmosphere if communication isn't handled carefully."

~Expecting caregivers to understand and communicate like office people is a mistake. They may see three to four different people and go to different places to do their work every week. They have to be more adaptable, and have more variables in their work day, than any office person you know.

~They are paying YOUR salary—please never allow

your office staff to forget that. I will get rid of an office staff person for being rude or snide to a caregiver, because the caregiver truly does all the work.

✔ **Mutual respect is everything.** Respect is the biggest factor in caregiver etiquette—talking to them with appreciation and kindness, being careful how you express concerns, and respecting their feelings and time. Do not continually cancel a caregiver without giving him or her a coffee gift card, an hour of pay, etc. (See below—Incentives.)

✔ **Clarity: Be clear & direct. Do not manipulate. Do not be passive. (Sensing a trend here?)**

NO: "Umm, do you think you can go to Mrs. Brown on Saturday, is that okay? Yes? Okay, bye."

YES: "Mrs. Brown needs someone every Saturday from 8 a.m. to 4 p.m. Can you do that? Yes? Okay, get a PEN—and write down this address."

NO: "Hey honey, she says you are not on time."

YES: "You need to arrive a few minutes early. If shift starts at 8, we will pay for you to arrive at 7:45, because you cannot be late to our case."

NO: "Try it and see."

YES: "I need someone she can bond with and count on. If you like it, can you commit to being her permanent person for her whole schedule?"

NO: "It is an easy case, just give it a try."

YES: "She needs a lot of TLC. Be kind and anticipate what she needs. I think you are the best fit for her."

✔ **About "being late..."** If a caregiver was always late on a prior case, when you staff him/her on a new case, CLEARLY state that such behavior will be unacceptable on this new case: "You were late three times to Mrs. Jones. If I place you with Mrs. Smith and you are late *once* I will have to let you go."

Pro Tip: Clearly state what the pay rate is, and if it is higher or lower than the default (usual) pay scale, put it in writing—that it is for this client only, *and have your caregiver sign.* You don't want them to quit because pay is too low, or have them expect a higher rate on *all* cases.

✔ **Be kind and concerned.** Caregivers spend all of their time caring for others. They need a little kindness when being dealt with on a daily basis, and you as a business owner need loyalty; and loyalty does not happen when you are unkind or inconsiderate.

✔ **The Art of Listening = Success (or Failure).** Listen when a caregiver gives you spoken and unspoken clues.

> **As a Home Care Owner, you must learn to INTERPRET and read between the lines.**

Spoken: "My daughter/son just joined a sports team. I am so proud!"

Unspoken: This usually means that there will be days they are newly unavailable due to "game days." You need to ask that up front.

Spoken: "Mrs. Smith keeps changing her hours. You need to call Mrs. Smith."

Unspoken: Your caregiver is probably going to leave. This is a "light complaint" that will lead to big problems later.

Spoken: "Jenny at your office doesn't return my calls," "is rude," or "my paycheck is wrong."

Unspoken: Make sure you fix these issues, because caregivers gossip, and you will find your caregivers start talking to each other about complaints.

Spoken: "I am going to school for..."

Unspoken: Find out when, and the schedule. The sooner you know, the better off your preparations are for your client.

Spoken: "Mrs. Smith asked me to work outside of my scheduled hours."

Unspoken: You need to visit Mrs. Smith and politely make sure she understands to go through the office.

Spoken/Observable: Caregiver begins to come in looking disheveled.

Unspoken: Pull them aside, privately, and speak to them. Things could be going on at home.

Spoken/Observable: Your caregiver who is usually on time begins being late.

Unspoken: Pull them in and talk one on one—could be a new babysitter, a new second job, etc.

Spoken: Caregiver begins to ask for advances all the time.

Unspoken: Caregiver is not working enough shifts, and/or is in some kind of trouble.

Spoken/Observable: Caregiver is at the client's home when they are unscheduled—and it is not on their timesheet.

Unspoken: They are working off books and will probably steal your client.

Spoken/Observable: Caregiver is suddenly unresponsive to calls and texts.

Unspoken: Your caregiver has found another position. Place them on "Inactive" and leave them a final message to "call when they are *available to reapply.*"

Spoken/Observable: A caregiver no-shows to a case.

Unspoken: They are "going down the rabbit hole." They will blame it on a million things. If you want to give them another chance, fine. But the second time is no mistake — *let them go.*

✔ **Create a company culture of mutual respect.** Be kind when dealing with caregivers and office staff alike, and create a company culture of reciprocity and professionalism. I like staffers that listen to their caregivers and are personable and appreciative, as well as know how to keep healthy boundaries.

When you have a staffer that makes "friends" with his/her caregivers, then you run the risk of allowing unprofessional behavior to continue, favoritism, or any number of troubling circumstances that undermine the reputation of the company.

✔ **Be professional and have high expectations**.

Explain to clients and caregivers what your agency stands for, and what your service expectations are.

~When caregivers get riled up, ask them to calm down, then be quiet and *listen* to what they are saying.

~When a caregiver makes an error or gets a complaint, tell them what the error is in a kind manner.

~When a client complains, offer IMMEDIATELY to change caregivers, and make sure you keep great notes so anyone can access caregiver history. *DO NOT convince a client to keep a caregiver they do not want — they will begin to look elsewhere for care.*

"When your caregiver loves a client and goes

above and beyond—let the family know.
They will love you for it."

~If you have to give a discount based on caregiver behavior or lack of skill set, remove that caregiver. Remember, you are looking for longevity.

~The best match is a long term and mutually caring relationship, but caregivers cannot have clients concerned over their life situations, so remind your caregivers with problems to keep them private.

~There is NO lending/borrowing of money *ever* allowed (unless, as the owner, you want to pay it back—because caregivers never do). Make that clear to all caregivers and every client.

~There is NO bill paying, or writing of personal checks to caregivers.

~There is no gift giving unless it is signed off (in writing) by the office AND any family members involved in the care.

~There is no rudeness (even to office staff) allowed by your caregivers—get rid of them.

~Be willing to pass along a case that is not appropriate for your agency. A skilled need, for example, if you haven't been licensed for nursing.

✔ **When to convince, plead or beg!** *It is 4 p.m., and your caregiver has cancelled for their shift starting at 5 p.m. You are desperate. You are sweating. The client has no idea—*

what do you do?

~On weekends when staff is limited (see below), or after hours when you would like to sleep, it is also okay to beg.

~Offering more money is, as an owner, always my first course of action. I up the ante by $2 to $4. <u>For that shift only.</u>

~Alternately, I may offer a gas card or (small) gift card to their favorite store, or a coffee gift card.

~Depending on the circumstances, you may want to offer to give them the whole case if they do well.

> *"DO NOT convince a client to keep a caregiver they do not want—they will begin to look elsewhere for care."*

~Allow them to get overtime ***if*** they have already worked 40 hours that week.

~Do *not* get angry when they say no—just thank them for their time and move on to the next one.

~Offer to give them a ride.

~If it is a 12-hour shift, and they just take the first half, that buys you the time you need to staff the second half.

~Staff anyone (your third string caregivers are okay here)—and then explain to your client that it was an emergency.

✔ **How to deal with "There's no one left."** Here's another common scenario: *It is 4:15 p.m. on Friday and you have just gotten a call for a 24-hour, high dollar, around the clock case! Your staffers groan: "There is NO ONE LEFT!" They love to say this. It is the mantra.*

"I've called EVERYONE."

Don't buy it.

Pro Tip: Send out a mass text to set up the weekend care at $3 above your pay rate, and staff the case **through Tuesday night.** *Never leave a Monday morning shift open, or a Monday night.* Staffers come in from the weekend lazy, and problems happen Monday morning. But since you have offered "Emergency Pay," you will be able to staff the client quickly and efficiently.

~Another option is giving overtime to those great caregivers who have already worked 40 hours. You will spend more in staffers' OT than you will in caregiver OT.

✔ **Giving accolades, incentives and kudos.**

Remember: Anything a client says about your caregivers, they are saying about YOU. So let it be known company-wide if possible.

~Give Starbucks cards for kudos. (Letters from clients.)

~Always tell the caregiver when the client says nice things, and vice versa. When your caregiver loves a client and goes above and beyond—let the family know. They will love you for it.

When a client and caregiver are a great match, listen to the caregiver's impression of the client's needs so you can offer other services that you may have relationships with (medical equipment, home heath, etc.).

~Always do something special on paydays. Have cookies or snacks in the office and have a staff member available to chit chat with caregivers about their cases.

Bottom Line: Hold your caregivers in high regard. If you were a clothing store they would be your clothing, and you wouldn't manhandle the merchandise and expect it to sell.

Caregivers are who represent you as an agency. We call them our "*ABS Brand Ambassadors*" because they represent us both in the community and in the client's home. Everything we stand for, and everything we have promised, lies in the hands of our Caregivers.

CHAPTER 10
GROOMING

(What is it and why do it?)

Staying in control of your business and managing your reputation means everything to the longevity of your success.

The ability to create a *synergy* between your clients and office will determine whether or not you keep a case — or the caregiver keeps the case. You want the case to be YOURS. This helps you stay ahead of complaints, and beat the competition.

Lia's Story:
Why Grooming Is Essential

"I had a case that we had been staffing for months, 24 hours a day. Great billing hours; the caregivers were happy, the client was happy (we thought). It was a wonderful case. Then, after almost 8 months on the case, the children contacted me, horrified. They were leaving our agency — immediately! Why? Well, the house was filthy, laundry was piled up, there were cockroaches in this beautiful home, and

the clients (husband and wife) had huge BEDBUGS in their mattresses and sheets, visible to the naked eye! The clients had dementia. Imagine how I felt? My caregivers weren't doing ANYTHING but collecting a paycheck, and, because the case was quiet, I didn't 'groom it' or even visit after the first week.

We saved the case, but I had to replace all of the furniture, hire a cleaning company, get rid of half of the caregivers and REMIND my supervisors to visit the case. GROOMING is essential for client safety, reputation, brand consistency, quality control and caregiver supervision."

~~~

1. So what is "Grooming"?

Grooming is the act of combing through the services you are providing, ensuring that the experience of Home Care is not only a great one, but that client and caregiver are a good match, and that the Service Expectations are being met. Grooming a case takes many forms, requires consistency and different types of personnel.

2. The Players Involved

✔ Care Managers

At ABS, your Care Managers are your Marketing and Sales Personnel. We have found that just having Sales and Marketing Reps, in this industry, does not work out well—they need to be able to identify with the clients' needs and handle issues on a high level in order to sell our services.

The Senior and Home Care industry is different from many industries because we are not "Direct Sales." We are creating (and selling) Relationships of Trust, and that means your top sales people must be trustworthy when given a Referral.

~They have to remember what is going on in the case.

~They often have their cell phone numbers on business cards, so they are the first person the client or their family calls.

~They are the "Assessment People," so they are making the original promise for great Service.

~They are the ones who close the deal.

~Care Managers are the only staff members who have FIRSTHAND knowledge of the client and their family's expectation of services.

It is their job to *impart* that consistency to your staff members, so everyone is aware and can provide services accordingly.

"We have found that just having Sales and Marketing Reps, in this industry, does not work out well—they need to be able to identify with the clients' needs and handle issues on a high level in order to sell our services."

✔ Care Coordinators

Care Coordinators are, for ABS, either highly skilled Caregivers (with knowledge of Hoyer lifts and protocols) or Licensed Vocational Nurses. They are presentable, professional and can stand in for Care Managers.

~They oversee the Referral Source Relationship by dropping brochures, checking on the clients and reporting back to referral sources. They also conduct Client Visits.

~For Registry Staffing, they are the ones who oversee that book of business.

Care Coordinators also:

~Get the weekly schedules.

~Check on completion of paperwork.

~Ensure that the facility/community is up to date on their billing/collections.

~See if there are other shifts to be obtained.

~Verify that the caregivers are meeting client expectations.

~Walk in new caregivers and orient them to the client's care needs.

~Report back to the office regarding client concerns or care concerns they may need to enforce in the future.

~Regularly reassess client needs to determine whether more or less service requirements are needed.

~Work the weekends.

~Must be detail oriented.

~Control Care Manager burn out.

Pro Tip: Beat your competition by having your Care Coordinators in certain buildings and marketing—*on the weekends.*

Care Coordinators truly manage your care and allow you to comfortably sell the fact that your company has 24-hour-a-day/7 days a week availability of office staff.

✔ Field Supervisors

These are your lowest level of Care Control and Client Management, but come from your roster of Top Tier caregivers. They must always be exceptional caregivers—professional and patient.

They do NOT sell. They do Client Visits and Walk Ins for new caregivers or new clients.

~By doing the Walk Ins and Opens, Field Supervisors ensure the quality of the match between client and caregiver.

~Field supervisors are directly over the caregivers we send out.

~They must know the company, and be pro-company all the way: They are your Company Ambassadors.

Field Supervisors must also:

~Be able to speak with caregivers regarding *company culture.*

~Still be providing care to at least one client so they maintain integrity in their visits, and can honestly relate to other caregivers.

~Be willing to jump in and do anything. Like your Care Coordinators, they may give rides or step in for a few hours on a case.

~Inspire confidence and security to both clients and caregivers.

~Be detail oriented, because they are placing client/caregiver notes in your system.

~Work the weekends and about 25 hours per week.

"Field Supervisors must know the company, and be pro-company all the way: They are your Company Ambassadors."

✔ Compliance/Staffing Personnel

This is an inside office person whose task is to maintain contact with family and clients *by phone.*

~They call clients to ask how things are going. (Weekly is preferable, but as you grow, every two weeks is acceptable.)

~They utilize the Database Dashboard and place notes in the system under "Client" and attach to caregiver files.

Compliance/Staffing Personnel also:

~Report client complaints and caregiver concerns to all staff.

~Obtain general information, as well as Scheduling changes.

~Report back verbally to family if there are any care concerns.

~Make requested scheduling changes.

~Set up additional Care Coordinator/Field Supervisor visits.

3. Best Practices for Grooming

Bottom Line: Do not promise something if you cannot deliver it.

Grooming costs money, because the personnel are Quality Assurance, not driving business or providing care.

✔ **Whose job is it to run the show?** In the beginning of your business, the owner or staffing manager should take on this role.

~This can be done when the company has 15 or less clients.

~If you have a Nurse on staff, they can take the role of Care Coordinator and bring a higher level of quality to your agency.

✔ **Timing or frequency:** Pick one day a week where they (or you) go out in the field and see the clients being serviced.

✔ **What are the benefits of grooming?** Grooming creates a bond and high trust levels with referral sources and client family members.

Grooming also gives caregivers a sense of security, and lets them know that they truly have the support of an agency and are part of a team.

✔ **Company Protection: What to look out for generally on grooming visits.** Are there any hints that may suggest the client is unsatisfied? Ask family members for any concerns you can focus on.

~Ask what the caregiver has been doing RIGHT.

~Always let the caregiver know of any compliments.

Look for:

~Caregiver complaints regarding payroll or staffing.

~Any procedures that are not company policy (coming by off schedule, calling on the phone).

~Any questionable behavior (disappearing, borrowing money, etc.).

~Valuables that are not locked or in a safe place and remove them (give them to family).

~Fall risks/safety issues.

~Is the food in the refrigerator fresh?

~Is the client clean?

~Is the house clean?

~Are there adequate supplies and is the client healthy?

> *"Always let the caregiver know of any compliments."*

✔ **Going deeper: Troubleshooting on grooming visits.** First off, do not always assume that a caregiver needs to be replaced if there are concerns. Listen carefully:

~Understand the diagnosis.

~Understand the dynamic.

~Be willing to train the caregiver.

~Keep the confidence of the client and the family, but be aware of their concerns.

~Wait until the caregiver leaves the job site before discussing any disciplinary action or negative feedback.

~Do not talk *about* the caregiver *in front of* the caregiver.

~Always let family members know when you are going to the client's home.

~If the client is alert and aware, make an appointment with them.

~Remember that everything must be documented and dated for client and company safety.

~Be prepared to let the caregiver go if absolutely necessary.

Pro Tip: Clients like to talk. So make sure your compliance person, and your field supervisors, have adequate time to remain in conversation during their visits.

✔ **What to encourage:**

~Encourage "kudos" or written statements regarding a

particularly good caregiver.

~Ask for *Yelp!* or other reviews, both online and locally.

~Find out other information that is not in the current care plan and update the current care plan accordingly, alerting all team members.

~Make sure the caregivers are Brand Ambassadors: Dressed professionally with a great attitude.

Always be respectful of caregivers and clients alike when you are in the home.

The Home Care Bible

CHAPTER 11
TROUBLESHOOTING

(Problems, Complaints, "Issues," Oh, My!)

1. Ground Rules for Troubleshooting

Different employees within your Agency will handle problems in varied ways, and as you grow, you need a clear protocol for how they are to be handled, so everyone not only "stays in their lane," but so they are also effective and don't "Band Aid" a problem over and over again, to the point of losing a client—or worse, your reputation—or even get sued.

> *"What most owners don't understand is EVERYONE has complaints and problems. How you handle them differentiates your agency."*

Further: All employees are *mandated reporters* regarding complaints of abuse or other serious issues, but they should never come to any conclusion without first notifying the CEO.

Lia's Story:
Clearly State Your Chain of Command

I had a manager who hired a great caregiver and, before her background check came back, she was placed with a client who loved her. Her background check then came out, showing that she had charges for heroin use/possession — as well as other various drug charges. The manager chose not to tell me (the CEO) because, over time, when she had told me about other issues, I had told HER to handle them — without truly listening or establishing a procedure or protocol.

Nonetheless, the manager claims that, after this particular background check came back, she was going to tell me the next day. But unfortunately, that very day, the caregiver was high, and got into a car accident with her 85-year-old client, who had dementia. The accident broke 12 bones in the client's body. The caregiver walked away without a scratch. The client's family sued our company for $1.2 million. It cost me over $60K to fight the lawsuit, and I made payments on the $250K settlement — all because my staffer/manager did not tell me, because I did not CLEARLY communicate the chain of command.

~~~

2. The Chain of Command

✔ **Caregivers/Nurses:** They should directly bring the problem to their immediate supervisor — this is the **staffing personnel.**

✔ **Staffing Coordinators:** Make sure the staffing coordinators KNOW they are the First Responders.

Staffing Coordinators must:

~Document all incidents.

~Make upper management aware of all incidents.

~Triage the complaint:

Is it serious?

Will it affect the company?

Does it affect the client?

Is there an immediate threat to health, safety or liability exposure – and, if so, what needs to happen NOW?

~Serious issues requiring immediate action: Staffing Coordinators must email everyone ASAP.

Examples: "The client is still driving after we leave," "I feel threatened by the adult son," or, "I feel sexually harassed." "This client has fallen." "I have hurt my back/arm/whatever." These are serious.

"Make sure the staffing coordinators KNOW they are the First Responders."

~Not serious: Staffing Coordinators are to place a message in the Call Center, but do not email everyone ASAP.

Examples: "I need to be off next Friday." "I cannot service this client due to change in schedule." "This client doesn't like Suzie." "The house is a mess." "The client's daughter is coming over tomorrow." *These should be placed in the Database Dashboard but not emailed to everyone.*

✔ **Field Supervisors:** Field Supervisors document and handle the smaller issues that the staffers are notified for. They also walk in caregivers to new clients and report issues that may arise.

Field Supervisors are the second level of "Triage."

Field Supervisors must:

~Document all incidents they are aware of.

~Notify the office via Supervisory Reports every time a client or patient is visited or a complaint is resolved.

~They are often called the "Band Aid" because they are limited in their problem solving approach by the incentives and compensation they can offer.

~They can hold the case together, but a secondary visit is recommended.

Field Supervisors basically handle anything that is a caregiver-related issue or change in service.

~"I need to be off next Friday." Field Supervisors walk in and train the replacement.

~"This house is a mess." Field Supervisors "drop in" and observe work conditions.

~The client has issues with a caregiver. Field Supervisor can relay those issues and express those concerns.

~The client has a complaint, but doesn't want to make a change. Field Supervisor will speak with both client and caregiver to gain a better understanding.

~The caregiver doesn't feel adequate to perform the client's needs. Field Supervisors train caregivers while on the job.

✔ **Care Managers.** Complaints are handled by Care Managers when:

~A referral source may become notified.

~The complaint may cause backlash to the company's reputation.

~The client is so upset that the case could be lost, or there is family member involvement.

Care managers also:

~Are your Sales/Marketing personnel.

~Have the polish to deal with family members.

~Need to go back and get ahead of client issues and

complaints with their referral sources so that they appear proactive.

~Are usually the ones that have assessed the case so they have a relationship with the client/family already.

Care managers are the final step before the owner.

Typical Care Manager complaints:

~Sexual Harassment. Removing the caregiver from the case; documentation; client and family intervention.

~Caregiver Theft. Taking a report; negotiating company repayment or facilitating Bond insurance.

~Client continuously making unreasonable demands. Speaking with family and client.

~Client has a complaint about office staff member. *Case Manager needs to bring it to the owner or CEO.*

~Client is unhappy with changes, or threatening to leave company — for any reason.

3. CEO/Owner — The Base of the Support Pyramid

As the owner of a NEWER agency, all concerns should be handled by you. It is easy to determine: If you do not have the levels of staff listed above, then insert yourself at the level that you have not yet employed. As a small or newer agency, your company reputation and growth rests on you, and how well you handle conflict and problems. What most owners don't understand is, EVERYONE has complaints and problems. How you handle them differentiates your agency.

I know we think of Burger King's slogan, "Have it your way" as the ultimate in customer service, but in Home Care that is not always the case.

Remember: Every complaint catches us off guard and places us on the defensive, so try to slow down your thought process.

✔ **Defend your caregivers or nurses.** A good rule of thumb is: "I have never understood her to say/do/be anything like that."

✔ **Make sure you have the whole story**. "Let me have a chat with the caregiver and see what her explanation is."

✔ **Test the severity of the situation.** A good question to ask is, "When would you like me to replace your caregiver?" Their response will indicate how bad the complaint truly is — if they say "no" or "not right away," then you need to determine if this caregiver needs to be removed at all.

✔ **Make an appointment to meet with the client.** (Either by phone or in person.)

✔ **Give a discount on service that was performed, but be careful.** (See Lia's Story, below.)

✔ Make sure you set very clear boundaries.

Lia's Story:
Handling "Constant Complainers"

*I have a client who called my Care Manager every other day about a caregiver saying or doing something. My care manager would run over and stand in while we chose another caregiver, or she would discount huge blocks of time. She would listen to the (drunken) daughter complain and whine. Now, this is a great case — over 16 hours a day, but my care manager was **overcompensating** for complaints that were real or imagined. I was losing time and money, and quite frankly, I was tired of hearing about it!*

So I began taking the calls.

In the past, the client's daughter would interview a caregiver, choose her over a regular that had been on shift, befriend the new caregiver, and then use their personal traits against them, to complain to us, and attempt to get a discount (as she had so many times before).

Now, when she called to complain, I listened. And listened. I did not speak, as she told me her caregiver had an "attitude" with her, and she therefore did not want to pay for the 7-hour shift.

I said I would replace the caregiver immediately — and she responded with, "No, I want to give her another chance." I explained that I could not conceivably refund the shift as, 1) she called after the shift had completed, and 2) by keeping the caregiver there, I would run the risk of refunding every hour she works if she makes the same mistake again.

I went on to say, "Let me speak with her. And, how about you agree to let me know AT THE BEGINNING of shift if it still is not working out, so I can replace her, and we see how it goes?" It worked. She doesn't complain as much, I have a Field Supervisor visit every two weeks, and we are still on the case.

Sometimes, some clients just need a little TLC.

~~~

✔ **Care Managers' job is to "sell care," so you must run interference at times.** Don't ever forget: Care Managers are ultimately sales people; they cannot handle major problems because they have to SELL, and that means they have to think your service is great! So remember to take the *constant complainers* off of their hands — and let them know afterwards how you have handled the complaint.

"If you do not have the levels of staff listed above, then insert yourself at the level that you have not yet employed."

✔ **Learn to know when "enough is enough."** Be willing to give up the client if you cannot adequately service them. A lot of CEO's and Care Managers, as well as staffers, think it is ANYTHING for the case. But if my service isn't great, my reputation will suffer, so I am always willing to let go of an unhappy client — *if I have done everything reasonable.*

Bottom Line: This philosophy must be communicated

out loud to your team, because staffers will begin to HIDE problems if they think you are going to blame them, and Care Managers will start bending over backwards, when, in some cases, clients can be better served by another agency.

✔ **Remember to remain calm and keep the lines of communication open**. No matter what, your whole staff should go through Customer Service training. We are dealing with very stressed out people in the BEST of times. Clients are paying to *feel better*, not to have a Band Aid placed over their concerns, or to be ignored.

The biggest issue in any company is communication, so make sure as you grow to ensure open lines between complaints systems — from the receptionist to the CEO — everyone must be on the same page.

CHAPTER 12
ALL THINGS MONEY

(Payroll, Billing, Collections, Margins
...and those other pesky little things that keep you afloat.)

For some, this chapter will be the most interesting. However, those are the financial people—who probably don't need this chapter at all! As a Caregiver turned Entrepreneur, this is the chapter that I needed to highlight, take notes on, and memorize; things that I am still learning to this day.

"Do not cut corners or pay under the table:
It will ALWAYS bite you in the end."

With all the changes in technology, at some point this chapter will be outdated, so if I reference specific programs, like "QuickBooks," please understand that it can be any "billing system." The same goes for payroll systems: They are your choice, *I am not recommending one over another.*

1. General Comments On Billing

Some rules of thumb to keep in mind:

✔ **Choose what works for you and stick with it.** If you are smart, you will find and set up a system that works forever. For me, I changed *billing* from monthly to bi-weekly — to now weekly — over the course of 18 years. I have changed *payroll* from bi-monthly to every other Friday.

Both the billing and payroll changes were major overhauls and I don't recommend this at all.

✔ **Know there is lag time between inflow and outflow.** Now, if you are doing your own payroll and billing and are just starting out, you will quickly see that money doesn't come in as fast as it goes out. In Home Care, we are constantly trying to "make ends meet" and get ahead of our income. One of the reasons for this is we pay in Real Time — which means, whether or not your CLIENTS pay you, your CAREGIVERS must be paid, causing the lag time.

✔ **"Leave it!"** In general, don't touch the money in your account. It may look like your profit is there, but ignore it, because at some point, you will need it.

Pro Tip: Clients and caregivers have one thing in common — they don't like change. So take a moment to review your own pros and cons behind the scenes, then move forward with confidence as you do your billing and payroll. Train them in what to expect.

Lia's Story:
Correct Errors With Kindness

When I first started my agency, it was just me doing everything, with a friend part-time taking in applications and answering phones. I would bill in my daughter's cramped bedroom on Sundays. We had no air conditioning, and I hate math, so I would be in there sweating like a pig while trying to be as accurate as I could.

I would DELIVER my billing. (I did that until I had 22 clients; then it got to be too hectic.) During this time, I had the opportunity to learn a very important lesson from one man: I was caring for his wife – a split shift; two hours in the morning, three hours at night.

This man said to me, after being on service for over a month, "If I tell you something, you won't back bill me for it, will you? I just feel so guilty, I need to let you know."

"Of course not!" I responded in my CEO, new owner, voice.

He said, "You have only been billing me for one shift. I owe you over $800, so can we start from today?"

I was not only embarrassed, I was grateful. I learned a valuable lesson, and it only cost me $800: When it comes to money, MISTAKES WILL ALWAYS BE MADE. YOU MUST STAY ON TOP OF IT. Double check your work.

I now have someone who does my billing, and – 18 years later – I still check her work from time to time. I also am very understanding when I find a mistake, you know why? Because that client's husband was very kind to me when I made a mistake. So learn from your mistakes, and, as you grow, treat your staff like this man treated me: kindly correcting an error.

~~~

"In general, don't touch the money in your account. It may look like your profit is there, but ignore it, because at some point, you will need it."

2. Specific Strategies for Billing

✔ **One option — billing in advance.** One of my friends who owns another agency is really smart — she actually bills in ADVANCE — which does several things in addition to the obvious (having the money for payroll):

~It keeps clients from changing their schedule.

~It keeps billing mistakes to a minimum, because you are billing based on numbers REQUESTED, not actuals, so clients understand when there is an issue. They do not understand when they are billed after service, because they THINK caregivers and timesheets are all magically synchronized in perfect timing, but they are not; *and billing errors exist due to bad calendars and schedule changes not being recorded.*

~It allows you to get a grasp on caregivers who aren't on time or are no shows, because clients will notify you — they know you bill based on the requested schedule.

The cons to billing in advance are:

~You will make mistakes regardless; schedules are fluid and times change.

~You may pay based on the assumption that the hours were worked, and later find out they were not worked.

~You may MISS billable hours, because caregivers will work extra hours and clients will not notify you, so you catch them later, and now you are "supplemental billing."

~Clients (and people in general) do not like to be billed BEFORE work is completed, so it can be a hard sell.

~If a client passes away or cancels services, you either need a very strong "no refunds" policy, or you will be cutting a lot of reimbursements, and I don't like that part.

"(L)earn from your mistakes, and, as you grow, treat your staff like this man treated me: kindly correcting an error."

✔ **Another option: Billing bi-weekly (every two weeks).** Two or three of my friends who established bill every two weeks. This works for a few reasons:

~In our industry, many times you have a *Third Party Payor* source (an adult child, fiduciary, or insurance) who tends to take their time when paying.

~Writing checks and paying bills is usually done on a monthly basis for most of us, so two weeks is closer to what people prefer.

~You have the time to get the EXACT billable hours from your caregivers because you bill around pay periods, so everything is turned in.

The cons to billing bi-weekly are:

~When someone gets behind in billing, they are REALLY behind, and only those with a nice cushion can afford that.

~There are often billing disputes, and two weeks is a long time to have to research and produce accurate records for when you need the income.

~When clients pass away, everything goes into probate, and the wait can be up to one year.

~If a client cancels you have to pay them back a lot of money.

~It can be a large amount of money if a client has 12 or 24 hours, and for me, it is easier to swallow an elephant one small bite at a time, meaning they may end services after seeing one large two week bill, but broken down it seems much more manageable.

✔ **A third option: Billing weekly.** I currently bill weekly. This works for me for a few reasons:

~I pay every other Friday, so there is a SLIM hope that

I will have adequate funds for payroll.

~I catch errors in hours a lot quicker, because clients are billed at the end of their week. (I bill Friday through Thursday — sent out on Thursday.)

~My collections or problem payors are caught very quickly.

~I am out less money when someone passes away.

~The errors, or issues, clients have are on a smaller scale, because it is only one week of mistakes.

~I can stay on top of my payroll and billing person a lot easier because I notice changes in billing levels.

~Did I mention I am NOT a mathematician? So it is easier for me to gauge company profitability on a smaller scale.

The cons to billing weekly are:

~If caregivers have to manually turn in time cards there may be errors in your billing if they are not in on time, and hours may have been adjusted.

~Clients do not like to write a check every week, so they let the bills pile up until THEY want to pay (which is usually every three weeks).

~Insurance and third party payors must be kept track of because they pay 30 to 60 days out.

~Overtime and other extra hours must be recalculated and "supplemental" billing does occur.

3. Forms of Payment to Consider

Pro Tip: Always encourage payment by ACH Bank Draft, or **Electronic Funds Transfer**. There are many companies that do this. Some, like Vanco Payment Solutions, charge approximately $6 per transfer, which is very inexpensive.

~Remember — **credit card charge fees** are anywhere from 2.5%-5% of your transaction, so you have to place a **surcharge** on your clients or take the loss.

~**Checks** are soon (I hope really soon) going to be a thing of the past, but in the 21st century, many people still pay their bills with checks. I recommend you charge a **"Transaction fee"** of at least $5.00 per payment. Discourage checks, mainly because you are not in control of when you receive payments.

Bottom Line: Drop off billing when you are starting out — it is the best way to stay in touch with your clients and on top of your services and reputation. *It also gets you paid a lot faster, because clients look forward to the visit and tend to pay with you there.*

4. Payroll

There are really very few hints to payroll. But there is one thing to remember — *when you are dealing with money, people can get very emotional, and emotional people sue. Labor lawsuits can cost money, even if you AREN'T in the wrong.* So:

✔ **Pay correctly and know your labor laws**. Especially about split shift pay, per visit pay, mileage, and termination and final pay. Do not cut corners or pay under the table: It will ALWAYS bite you in the end.

✔ **Outsource Payroll.** Unless you are an accountant, find a great payroll company — ADP, PAYCHEX, ECHECKS — or use QuickBooks (or another software program like that).

~The biggest problem I see when people do their own payroll is filing your 941 taxes — or your state taxes.

Example: Your actual numbers for payroll are $45K. Taxes on that $45K are $8K. A payroll company would charge you $53K and file your taxes. If you do your own payroll, you would have the option of filing every three months if you choose to, but what if something comes up? And you don't have $24K in the bank (three months' worth of taxes/$8K). So what do you do? And how does it feel taking big chunks instead of little pieces?

Bottom Line: I am a fan of getting used to the larger bill, and being covered, instead of remembering to give Uncle Sam a large chunk every three months. But the choice is yours.

~**PEO** — Professional Employer Organizations; they are your All-In-One service. They charge an "administration fee" and do all of your payroll, usually your Human Resources, as well as your Worker's

Compensation insurance.

If your Worker's Compensation insurance is high, I recommend a PEO. If not, I highly recommend you keep everything separate. The biggest thing is that they take it all out at once, so there are no pesky calculations or audits from your Worker's Comp company that end up in high bills due to mistakes.

✔ **Remember to pay a decent salary, and pay your employees on time, BEFORE you pay yourself.**

Sounds like common sense, but many owners will pay themselves and have employee paychecks bounce. Caregivers and Nurses talk; and it is a small industry, so your reputation could be tanked with a few "held checks" or "incorrect payroll" incidents, when employees interview at other agencies and tell them about how you do business.

So the name of the game is: *1. Labor Law Knowledge (be willing to call and check for accuracy), 2. High Integrity, and 3. Don't Be Greedy and Squeeze Your Employees.*

THEY are your business. Treat them well and they will be with you for years. I have employees that I hired over 18 years ago that still work for me and know how much I care for them. It is THEM, not me, who create my reputation.

5. Your Salary

One of the things new owners don't know is WHEN they get paid, and then HOW they get paid.

Lia's Story:
Play the Long Game and Make Payroll

I used to see money in the bank and take it – if it looked like I had made $22,000 that month I would pay myself $15,000. In my early years, I wrote a check for my first Lexus at $35,000.00. I would see an "extra" $75,000 in my account and I would purchase a rental property. This was awesome! I looked up one day, and I owned three or four houses and some nice cars.

But 10 years had gone by, and I was still struggling to make payroll, and I PERSONALLY didn't have much money in the bank. Then I hit 50 years old, and realized that my office staff was in better retirement shape than I was! So I had to start from the beginning. I sold the houses and placed the money back into the company and into my savings. I began to have Peace of Mind – AND make Payroll!

~~~

✔ **If you are a sole owner, you are only** *stealing from yourself* **if you move money.**

✔ **All of the money in the bank is yours, and it works better if you save.**

✔ **Get yourself a good 401K or IRA, and be careful about vesting with employees in the beginning.** I did this, and the 401(k) company took money FROM me, because I was too highly compensated in comparison to my staff. So they TOOK from my distribution and GAVE to the others—EEEEEKK! It was all MY money, so I ended that very quickly!

Today, the programs are so much better, so find a good one and offer it to your staff, and take part in it, while building your *own* IRA.

✔ **Buy what you NEED, not what you want, in your first five years in business**, and begin to pay off things like houses and cars to place you in position to retire.

Pro Tip: When you are billing $15K per week, pay yourself (on payroll) $3,500 per month and utilize that formula moving forward. (When you are billing $30K per week, your salary doubles to $7,000 per month.)

You'll begin to feel "comfortable" at about $60K per week, which usually, if you follow my methods, happens in about 3-4 years. This is $3.120M per year, and you are on payroll earning $10.5K per month. (Remember, it is being taxed—this allows for your taxes at the end of the year to sting less. Also, see owner's draws, below.)

6. Owner's Draws, Reimbursements, Company Credit Cards

These are all ways to capitalize on the lower tax rates.

✔ **Owner's draws are taxed at a lower rate than payroll taxes.**

Beware: Owner's draws should always be less than 60% of your salary. (I didn't learn this until the EDD audited me and I ended up paying almost $70K in taxes. My CPA had given me BAD advice—saying you could take Draws instead of Salary—but there are specific rules for this.)

For example, I pay myself $100,000 a year on payroll with all applicable taxes paid (anywhere from 22%-35% **depending on your state**). I can draw 60% of that, so $60,000 can be disbursed to me in owner's draws, taxed at about 15%. Pretty simple.

✔ **Reimbursements and when to use the Company Credit Card.**

Your taxes become quite heavy when you have incorporated your business. (I prefer an S Corp, not an LLC, but the choice is yours. I feel more protected with an S Corp, if done correctly; but I have heard different opinions.)

Use your company credit card for:

~Gas Monday through Friday.

~Company furniture.

~Meals.

~Christmas gifts, bonuses, gift cards and other employee gifts. (Do not give cash—that looks like a profit, not an expense.)

✔ **Profit Sharing is the term used whenever you disperse funds from your company to yourself or others and they ARE TAXED.** When I disperse and expense funds over $600, I need to issue a 1099 tax form so that I can use them as a write off for the company. If I don't, they are considered INCOME, and I am taxed on them instead of the employee.

"(T)here are as many ways to figure margins as there are fingers and toes."

7. Financial Tips on Making Payroll, Keeping Collections Low and "Margins"

So I explained that I wasn't a financial guru, right? Well, good — this is the simple answer for those of us who are, ahem, challenged just a tad financially; or for those of us who "like to keep it simple."

✔ **Margins**: A great rule of thumb is to pay half of your billing amount. That can get harder as you begin to hire nurses at $28 per hour, yet the market will only bear a $45-an-hour charge. But with caregivers, it is a bit easier: If I am paying $13, then my goal is $26. So mainly I stay between $24-$26, and that way I am sure that, even as a franchise system, there is a level of *build out* for my 5% which allows a reasonable **margin** for myself. Now, there are as many ways to figure margins as there are fingers and toes.

~One way to calculate margins: Pay Rate x .55 = Y, plus the Pay Rate.

Take what you are paying and times it by .55 plus the pay rate; and then add that to the pay rate.

Example: I am paying $12 per hour x .55 = 6.6 + 12 =

$18.60. That is the high end (with taxes at 25% + overhead, insurances, staff, etc. at 30%), so the caregiver is COSTING me $18.60. If I am charging $20, then I am only clearing $1.40. Not good.

$$(\$12 \times .55 = 6.6) + 12 = \$18.60$$

$$\$20 - \$18.60 = \$1.40$$

Pro Tip: If you want a larger piece of the market share, don't "undercut" — offer "discounts."

When I started my company, I wanted to GRAB business and gain market share so I UNDERCUT — I took less margins for a larger piece of the business, and that worked. People like lower costs (hence Wal-Mart over Macy's). The problem is I became KNOWN for lower costs, and it took me YEARS to change my reputation to one of Quality over Price. So if you want to steal market share — offer DISCOUNTS — not low price. You will be locked in as "the cheapest agency," and that is hard to change.

~Another way to calculate margins: Bill Rate minus Pay Rate = Y, divided by Bill Rate.

Subtract your pay rate from your bill rate, and divide it by your bill rate again.

Example: I am paying $12, and I am billing $23, so 23 - 12 = 11 divided by .23 = 47.82% gross margin.

$$(23-12 = 11) \,/\, .23 = 47.82\%$$

Hard to understand? I told you so, and I have been mentored for over 10 YEARS on this stuff by one of my administrative mentors. (See Chapter 14 regarding Mentors.) **Yet I still try to maintain the standard of paying half of what I bill.** (Example: Pay $12, bill $24.)

Generate your reports from QuickBooks or your other billing and financial software.

> *"A great rule of thumb is to pay half of your billing amount."*

✔ **Monthly P&L (*Profit and Loss*) reports.** The Home Care business requires monthly P&L's. You can do this one of two ways:

~**General Report**: The general report is based on sales and bills, etc. for the month. This is the amount of money you SHOULD have.

~**Actuals Report**: The "Actuals" is a *cash accrual* report. This is the money you actually do have based on deposits and payments received. Some months will be higher due to getting large past due payments, and some months will be lower due to outstanding collections.

~These reports are done monthly so you can track spending and billing hours then translate that to income in a manageable way.

✔ An *Open Invoice* report should be run weekly to stay on top of collections.

Bringing us to our next topic:

✔ **Collections.** You do not want to get more than 14 days out on private clients, 60 days out on insurance, and no more than 30 days out on registry.

~What is your recourse for non-payment?

Calls, visits, and pulling care, are your recourse — before you hire a collection agency.

~Remember, we like bills in SMALL chunks. When you allow someone to get two or three bills behind, it is a larger check to write and it becomes harder to collect, so do yourself a favor and *make that call after the first bill.*

Pro Tip: Never send a second bill without the unpaid portion of the last bill on it. You are wasting paper. If someone is charged $300 per week and they are three weeks behind, why send ANOTHER $300 bill?

Send a $900 bill. That way, they are on the same page as you are. Bills may get misplaced and clients tend to pay one or two, and skip three and four.

"(R)emain consistent in your pay rate or all employees will become competitive and confused."

✔ **Stay on top of payroll**. Do not over-hire *office staff* because you are busy. Make sure you can afford it, and that you are going to maintain that level for the long term. If it is just a "spike" in billing, roll up YOUR sleeves (yes, yours—the owner's) and help out, until you are SURE you are going to maintain the billing hours to pay another salary.

✔ **Raises vs. Bonuses**. Don't start giving raises all over the place. A bonus structure works better because they revolve around your billing hours, so build in bonuses when you hire staff members. And even with caregivers, pay a higher rate for a long distance case, or for short hours, but otherwise remain consistent in your pay rate or all employees will become competitive and confused.

All staff talks, so if you are paying one person slightly higher—or a lot higher—than another, you will have to justify it, or deal with the feelings of resentment that come along with it, and this will lower caregiver and staff morale.

Bottom line: *Payroll must be met, and bills must be paid, so collections must be done, and a tight system is the best way to do business.*

CHAPTER 13
GROWING THE BUSINESS
YOU'VE BUILT

(Who to hire, and when.)

1. The Receptionist

The receptionist is always your first hire. So many Franchise Partners of mine, and even friends that found start-ups, like to hire a Marketing person first. They prefer to sit as opposed to build. There are so many reasons I hired a receptionist (a.k.a. *All Things Office* person) first:

✔ **I control the look and feel of my company and my reputation in the Marketplace.** As the Owner, I need to be *out in the field promoting my company.*

~There are a lot of days when the phone doesn't ring and sitting is a waste of time—and MY time is valuable.

~I need to always hire caregivers and nurses and I

cannot do that from the field. I need someone on the front end to process the applicants and coordinate the interviews while I am either out in the field *or* in an interview.

~Even if the receptionist only works part time to begin with, answering my phones for only half of the day means a break for me while I am meeting referral sources.

~It is less expensive to hire a part time receptionist than it is to hire a marketer.

~It is EASIER to TRACK a receptionist than it is to track a marketer.

Pro Tip: A good receptionist will turn into your first staffer, and you will want one of those faster than you think!

✔ **Six months in:** Your receptionist should have a $1 pay bump and is now your staffer. And now you and she/he should be sharing On Call, after hours availability.

2. Next Up: Your Junior Marketer

Your second hire should always be your Junior Marketer.

✔ **You know you're ready for a junior marketer when you have established yourself in the marketplace.**

~Your billing is no less than a steady $4,000 PER

WEEK.

~You know your referral sources.

~You have a Referral Source List with addresses, contact names and current emails.

✔ **Your Jr. Marketer is usually and should be a caregiver;** one that either looks great and sounds great and/or is a little arrogant or bossy; and is either from your roster, or a person from the outside.

"(A)s long as my billing remains at $100K or above, I buy lunch every Friday for the office staff to the tune of $100 per week."

~If you are smart and hire a caregiver, they can double as a Quality Control "Field Supervisor."

~Caregivers know the lingo and are more easily trained to do assessments.

✔ **Paying your Junior Marketer.** Your first Jr. Marketer is probably paid between $14-$16 per hour and works about 24 hours per week.

~Caregivers are less than "Marketers," who generally want $50K or more per year. (Hint: YOU are not even getting paid that yet.)

~They are spreading your brand and dropping brochures off; visiting new clients and checking on your service.

~The pay should include a SIMPLE bonus plan—either 2% of first two weeks of sales—or, $20 for cases that are 20 hours, $40 for cases that are 20-40 hours and $60 for up to 56 hours (8 hrs. x 7 days), and $100 for all hours above 57 hours per week.

~You can do any variation of those two scenarios, but stay on top of it—because bonuses eat your margins and are only meant as incentives and to encourage a junior marketer's vested interest in company growth.

Lia's Story:
Creating a Vested Interest In Company Success

I once was giving an Operations Manager 3% of net profit. I was giving my Marketer 2% of net profit. Billing was getting 2% of collected receivables, and my staffers were bonusing based on numbers. I looked up and I was losing tons of money. Bonuses and percentages are paid on ESTIMATED net profit, because collections and receivables do not really factor in. So my staff was draining me dry!

Another company larger than mine was paying their marketers a small percentage for the LIFESPAN of the case. Crazy! The minute they brought in enough to make a good bonus continually, they stopped trying. Neither bonus structure worked.

~~~

Bottom Line: Currently, I bonus my marketers 2.5% of the first month of billing. This is a high number, but I pay it **once** and it is usually my first month's profit. When you get to operations or partnerships, your bonuses are based on Gross Net or Net Profits, but they should always be on ACTUAL CASH ACCRUED, because that creates a vested interest in making the company cash-solvent.

3. And Then There Were Three — The $25K Mark

At around $25K a week, you should streamline and have one staffer, one Jr. Marketer and you.

✔ **Your staffer should be the only full-time person other than yourself.**

✔ **Your Jr. Marketer should now be working 30 hours per week.**

✔ **You are doing on call and switching it up with your staffer.**

✔ **You should have a roster of 40-50 caregivers.**

"(Bonuses) should always be on ACTUAL CASH ACCRUED, because that creates a vested interest in making the company cash solvent."

4. The $50K Mark: Party of Six?

✔ **For every $50K a week you have in billing, you need to add another staffing support person, a part time Field Supervisor and a Billing and Payroll clerk.**

✔ **Any one or several of these positions can be you, as long as you want to do them.**

5. At The Three-Year Mark: Groom Your Leads

Begin grooming your leads when you hit about three years in. You will want to step back and create your company — a company that runs without you.

> *"Do not get involved in or allow gossip or negativity into your office. It will wreak havoc on company culture."*

✔ **The Office Staff:** Begin loosening the reins to see what staff does when you are working part time.

~Ensure that you are always available by phone, email or text.

~Have frequent meetings to check the temperature of your staff.

~Do not get involved in or allow gossip or negativity into your office. It will wreak havoc on company culture.

~Create a bonus-based system where everyone wins when business is good. (See previous section on how to determine bonuses.)

Pro Tip: I like to take a day or two off, and I know that can create resentment among employees who do all of the actual "work" within the company. So as long as my billing remains at **$100K or above,** I buy lunch every Friday for the office staff to the tune of $100 per week.

~At this point, they have already hit key bonus points and are $15K away from the next one.

~It keeps them feeling appreciated (and they are—I ADORE my inside staff).

~I remind my staff how grateful I am by, guess what? TELLING THEM! I let them know: I can be off, away from the office—because they are so good at their jobs. And it's true.

✔ **Stop micromanaging.** Remember, staff don't really LOVE a boss hanging over them; and staff don't function well with micromanagement.

Bottom Line: I used to micromanage until I hired a higher level employee/manager, and then they politely asked me to "stop helping." Ha ha! I was miffed. My ego was bruised. And then I became very PROUD, and I felt a huge weight lift off of my shoulders.

✔ **Support your staff with On Call Staffing.** For at least three weeks out of the month, you need an afterhours "On Call" staffing person to take the weight and stress of staffing off of your office personnel.

6. On Call: What Is It? How Do Your Hire For It? And…Why?

I like to say Illness and Injury don't take a vacation and they don't care about holidays; they happen while I sleep and they happen while I am awake. That is why this is the best business to be in. It is not a store where you pay money and when the doors close so does your earning potential. NOPE. Illness and Injury are always chugging along, and you have caregivers and nurses working night shifts, morning shifts, Christmas Day shifts—and all of it is making you money. But what about when you DON'T want to answer the phones?

That is when On-Call comes in to play. It is also called After Hours Staffing, or Emergency Services. Many agencies will just go to Voice Mail after hours.

Well, no. For weekends and from 5 p.m.-8 a.m. you need someone answering your phones. In the beginning, that will be YOU for your first $3-5K a week in billing.

~It helps you stay on top of Staffer mistakes (people not getting correct information, clients not being told who is coming).

~It helps you recognize Bad Apples on your caregiving staff (late cancellations, problems while on shift, no call, no shows).

✔ **But On Call becomes a full-time position all in itself, and the pay rate depends on your state and your laws**.

~If your staffer is in California and does On Call, they should be a salaried personnel or they get paid hourly overtime.

~If it is just an afterhours person remaining *only after*

hours—in some states they can be independent contractors. But in others they are paid hourly or a set fee.

~On Call can go straight to the on-call phone or through an on call service.

~Straight to a phone means that someone can get a live voice at any time, but it also means there is very little tracking capability.

~Service will provide you with a call log telling you the calls that have come in.

~Either way the choice is yours, but you need to have an on call service if you want to be professional.

7. Caregiver Appreciation—Ongoing

✔ **Remember your Field Staff and how hard they work. (See Chapters 1 through 4.)**

~Send out birthday cards monthly for everyone working who has a birthday in that month.

~Have cookies or treats in the office on paydays.

~Make sure there is always someone (usually your least busy staffer) to listen and chit chat when caregivers come in.

~Your caregivers are your Brand Ambassadors. The way you treat them is the way they will treat and respect you and your clients.

"Kid gloves and lots of love"
is the saying we use.

~They are always caring for others, so you have to care for them.

✔ **Systems you can put in place to keep your caregivers "networked in":**

~Create a newsletter highlighting one caregiver a quarter or month.

~Create a Facebook page just for them.

~Have raffles for thanksgiving and other holidays and give out gift cards.

~Hold quarterly or monthly in-services or education seminars for those that want to attend.

~Send out mass letters thanking them, or reminding them of special things.

Pro Tip: Sell branded uniforms at a discount rate so they look professional.

~Weed out bad apples quickly.

"Your caregivers are your Brand Ambassadors. The way you treat them is the way they will treat and respect you and your clients."

7. General Tips

✔ **Keep your office environment cheerful and upbeat, and maintain a climate of mutual respect.**

This point has been restated throughout the Guide: Observe office staff-caregiver interaction closely, and make sure the office staff are treating the caregivers with kindness and respect.

Bottom Line: At 18 years in, I have hired and fired more than 50 office staff members (not counting caregivers) and I am *just now* getting it right. Hopefully you will read this book and get it right from the beginning.

The Home Care Bible

CHAPTER 14
BEST PRACTICES: THE MENTOR

(Excerpted from Smart Steps to Big Dreams)

1. Mentors: Find one

✔ **Do not expect them to hang out with you.** They are busy. Much busier than you are.

✔ **Do not expect them to tell you where they get business.**

✔ **Do not expect them to drop wisdom on you.**

At this point, you may ask: *"Well, Lia, what good is a mentor to me if I can't hang out with them and ask them all of my questions about building a home care business?"*

Here's the answer:

✔ **Watch them, and then conduct yourself like them.** Are they sitting on any Boards? Are they in positions of power? Are they attending certain functions? *Follow in their footsteps.* That is how we get ahead.

"I have acquired integrity and a loyalty towards (my mentors) in this business because their value to me is not in dollars, it is in **sense***...and that is priceless."*

2. The section below is excerpted from my book, *Smart Steps to Big Dreams*, taken from the chapter on mentorship:

You are doing well, better than me, and I look up to you, so are you my Mentor? That depends on *who I am*. We tend to think that we can find or ask someone to mentor us, they'll say "yes," then we lay at their feet, they give us pearls of wisdom and—Presto—we are doing great!

We don't account for our own jealousy, defensiveness, inability to execute, and our "mentor's" schedule. Eventually, we resent our mentor; they don't return our calls when we want them to, we are not "besties," they don't give us the time of day, or we start being in *competition* with our mentors—and let me help you out with something: A *true* mentor can smell a lack of integrity from a mile away.

Ask yourself:

1) Am I comfortable enough to ask for help?
2) Do I have my own circle of support?
3) Do I have integrity? (Am I still gossiping, fearful, needing accolades?)
4) Am I humble enough to allow for direction?
5) Do I know what I am looking for in a mentor?

When I started in this business, I had a mentor. She was harsh, she was blunt, but she was successful, and she helped me by using my company. Her name was Kathy. She owned her own agency and she was really smart. She gave me business and I supplied her with caregivers. She would throw me suggestions like how to handle my accounts and we hung out, marketing together, and she had been in business five years longer than me. And then things changed. At a certain point, I needed a GM, and her staffing person (who was a nurse) applied for the job. I asked her if it was okay, and she said yes, so I hired him. I wouldn't understand the distance it created between Kathy and me for many years to come.

You see, Kathy wasn't a *mentor*, she was a *colleague* — a friendly competitor — because I wasn't ready for a mentor yet. Today, I have two mentors. Neither one of them give me business, unless they have to (smile), and I wouldn't dream of hiring someone who worked for them, and neither one of them would have trusted me ten years ago. (One still says, "Can I trust you with this?" And of course she can, but she is still leery.)

Because they have watched me around the community, and they respect what I have accomplished, there is no doubt that I am the "baby" (both financially and knowledge-wise) in the circle.

"You have to be content and confident in your business to truly acquire a mentor, and the reason it takes so long is because you have to WATCH for years to determine

what traits and qualities you want to align yourself with, especially if it is in the same industry."

I obtain mentors because of their knowledge base or other traits, NOT because of what they can do for me, or I for them. We're actually on different trajectories.

One of my mentors is literally a selfless servant to home care. She flies to DC and Sacramento and teaches, is on committees, and she has the most integrity I have ever experienced in this business. She is incredibly successful, with a 30+ year agency that her mother created, and she is as far from my background as you can get, but what am I learning from her?

How to stand up to people in this industry, how you can have integrity AND be successful when you do the right thing, also how to save my money and stop spending on frivolous things. When she speaks, I eat it up and listen.

My other mentor opened his company a few months after I opened mine, but honestly he is one of the financially smartest men I have experienced in this industry. I have watched and asked questions, he has always been honest and open, and he has built his business two or three times larger than mine, in less time. We are not "besties," speaking on the phone every day or going out for drinks (although when we have time, we do get together), but if you were to speak badly about either one of my mentors I would set you straight, and probably not engage with you again. I have acquired integrity and a loyalty towards them in this business because their value to me is not in dollars, it is in *sense*...and that is priceless.

"Carry yourself with integrity and respect, because one day, you might be the mentor that someone is looking for."

You have to be content and confident in your business to truly acquire a mentor, and the reason it takes so long is because you have to WATCH for years to determine what traits and qualities you want to align yourself with, especially if it is in the same industry. That is very tricky, because in my industry (home care), everyone is competition, and I have to align myself with those whom I do not want to compete with. That takes growth and is challenging on my part. I also need to have an integrity level that my mentors can respect. I cannot be needy, or not successful, as that is uncomfortable to people.

Pro Tip: It is easier if you have a mentor in another industry; they don't mind sharing their knowledge because you will never use it against them, and they usually are much less complicated relationships.

Learn the difference between friendly competitors and mentors.

When you first start out, you need *friendly competitors*, people who are on the same level with you. With friendly competitors, I keep my guard up, but can ask various questions, like how do you do payroll? Where do you get your caregivers? Let's hang out; let's sit together, those types of things.

With a *mentor*, we actually learn more by WATCHING than asking, and truly, most mentors don't have time to be interviewed or hang out, or answer inappropriate business questions. Mentors know you are in competition, and many times, with mentors, if you are in the same industry, business questions are literally off limits, which is why you have to be financially ready and at a business level you can relax in.

Bottom Line: Learn to understand the difference between Co-Learners or Friendly Competitors, and Mentors. Take the time to grow your business and work on your integrity level before seeking out a mentor in your own field. Understand that a mentor is not someone who owes you anything; they are someone who has capabilities beyond your scope of knowledge, and you'll need to respect that and do more listening than talking. Check your own confidence level and make sure you are not secretly competing with your mentor, because that will destroy your relationships, and lower the trust.

Remember that, the same way you are watching others, someone is watching YOU, so carry yourself with integrity and respect, because one day, you might be the mentor that someone is looking for.

CHAPTER 15
HOME CARE IN A NUTSHELL

(Some parting words of wisdom.)

Sometimes I truly believe that owning and running a home care agency has taught me more about MYSELF than any of the self-exploration courses of action I have taken. It has taught me how to treat people, and how to serve, while providing jobs for my community and giving me the incredible ability to make people safe in their homes — and at the same time affording me a lifestyle I could have only dreamed of.

1. A Brief Overview of My Business Philosophy

A Better Solution In Home Care, Inc. is my company, my passion, and I have grown it to be a major player in the industry.

I have franchised the concept, am licensed for Federal Medicare Billing, and have taken on two partners for these other methods of growth, but I am still very much in control of my home care agency — and I will never let it go.

Among all the success, I have had major failures and made incredible mistakes. If I could give you just one piece of advice, it would be to never give up, give 100%, don't get lazy, and don't rest on yesterday's success.

Home Care is a fluid business that creates a responsibility of its owners for people's lives, and how they are cared for by the people you hire. Take it seriously, take it personally, and you will never go wrong!

Caregivers & Clients are the only Stake Holders that matter.

2. Client Centric Care

When making the decision as to whether or not you want to choose being, or staying, in home care, there are certain levels of integrity and community that you must have in order to remain passionate about what you do, and create a successful and respected agency within your community.

A Better Solution In Home Care, Inc. has built its reputation on "Clients First, Caregivers Second, and everything else a Distant Third." We are not focused on OBTAINING clients, we are focused on placing the clients and the families that choose our agency first, in the line of how we treat and care for them. Seniors or the Medically Fragile individuals we deal with are our responsibility. We must be focused on keeping them safe and in a positive, protected environment.

That means they come first, before a caregiver, before even ME, as the owner. My clients take precedence. Why? *Because I can take care of myself, they cannot.*

"A good fit means that the case will run without incident and last a long time, all translating to easier and better business for me."

✔ **Clients don't live where we work. We work where they LIVE.** If you can place this as part of your mission, your philosophy, your true message to your staff, then everything will change. How you do business will change. *Why* you do business will change. Your level of gratitude will change, and then you can truly begin helping people, which is a much higher calling than just running a business. Client Centric Care is the ground work for everything A Better Solution stands for.

Lia's Story:
Don't Nickel & Dime Your Clients

We just received a client who was with another agency. I like the other agency. It has grown by leaps and bounds. The owners are very smart, and I love watching them rise. I have heard great things and admired them for several years. However, in speaking with this new client, I realized what their focus was: The client had to pay for every new caregiver to come and train for the position, at $65 per caregiver.

Now, that may not be much money, but after two caregivers didn't work out (no shows, etc.) and the THIRD caregiver *was coming for training, meaning another $65 fee, this client began to get fed up, wondering, "Why am I paying for the company to send the wrong fit?"*

The focus was financial. It may sound smart, but with a client telling friends and neighbors about the bad service, in the end it is detrimental.

~~~

✔ **As a Client Centric model, we don't nickel and dime our clients.** When training is needed, we send a care manager or field supervisor out, so they can train each new staff member, or you have them come in 30 minutes early at no charge. (See Chapters 10 and 11.)

The reason is twofold:

~A client is much more forgiving of changes in care staff when they receive a free service or the company takes on the burden; and

~It is *our agency's responsibility* to ensure qualified, trained individuals. That is our promise. So why would I charge the client to ensure a good fit? A good fit means that the case will run without incident and last a long time, all translating to easier and better business for me.

3. Have Integrity In How You Do Business and You Will Never Go Broke

Integrity in home care means always placing client care above financial gain. Now, am I saying give away free service? NO. Am I saying charge less? NO. What I am saying is: Charge what you're worth, and then go above and beyond. Have integrity.

✔ **If you know the caregiver you placed on a shift is not the greatest,** change him or her when you find someone better, or visit the client regularly so your caregiver can see the oversight and improve in his or her job.

✔ **Don't take clients you cannot service.** I have several agency owners that I like and do business with, and when I get a case—even a great money maker—that is out of my scope of care or my range of abilities (distance, skill level or requested type—i.e. a male caregiver who speaks Spanish, Yiddish, Japanese, Farsi, etc.), I call one of them and they provide the service needed.

My goal is to provide great care, not to stretch myself so thin that my reputation and capabilities suffer.

✔ **Tread carefully with supplemental staffing agreements.** I do a lot of supplemental staffing for smaller agencies, but I will not provide staff for under 8 hours, because under 8 hours is not worth the work load. In the past, I have provided supplemental staffing to other agencies that have stolen or approached my caregivers, and that causes problems. So I only staff for a handful of agencies.

~You have to TRUST who you work with, because the gain of a few dollars is not worth the loss of a great caregiver.

Pro Tip: I do not utilize "other" or supplemental staffing myself, mainly because I am too busy as an agency to oversee another agency's care that is given under my name, so I tend to just give the assignment or case away. It makes for great relationships and maintains my reputation as one who can find the referral sources and care anywhere.

I am known for my Business Integrity, and you cannot buy that. It is way too "expensive" to operate in a manner that lacks integrity, so do not poach referral sources or clients entrusted to you by other agencies.

"It is way too 'expensive' to operate in a manner that lacks integrity, so do not poach referral sources or clients entrusted to you by other agencies."

✔ **Always provide the BEST service for the client, not the service they "want."** Clients and their families have a tendency to look at *Cost* over *Care* — so if you assess a client who is bed ridden and the family says they want two hours of care, you know that is not the "best service for the client." *Explain to the family that it is unsafe.*

If they are financially challenged, find community service options for them, and provide the BEST service of your ability.

Everyone that comes into our lives once we begin working in the home care/senior field needs assistance or help or advice for some loved one or another. This will not always translate to dollars for you, but it is the business we are in. Your mindset must be one of service and assistance, of doing the BEST you can for everyone that seeks your care, and always telling them the TRUTH about their care needs.

Bottom Line: Whether or not they decide to take your suggestion is up to them, but owning an agency that truly serves others will give you an incredible feeling of satisfaction when you are honestly and carefully recommending and giving care advice to those that come to you.

4. Caregivers

Those who care for others must be handled with Special Care themselves.

Starting my career as a caregiver has given me a unique perspective on the behavior, characteristics, and abilities of our workforce. Being in business for over 18 years has also afforded me the ability to watch how others treat and see our caregivers, as well as how misunderstood they tend to be—by the very people who employ them—so a small "word to the wise" on this Stake Holder group is worth a recap:

Soon after the wonderful interview with the "Perfect Caregiver," you may find yourself angry and frustrated because he or she will not go to the client you need them to go to, or will not take the days and hours of certain shifts, or refuses to go back to another client, or maybe just doesn't show up!

I often hear new owners say, "Who Does that?!" when

discussing caregiver behavior.

"Great caregivers are like rare diamonds. They work and care for people because of their sensitivity and kindness, but when they are treated badly, that sensitivity can become surprisingly emotional or irrational, and that kindness can become aggressive, and sometimes it comes out of what you THINK is left field, but is actually from a lack of communication and listening that happens when people are treated as pawns."

✔ **Caregivers can be your best asset, biggest frustration, best friend, or a minefield that you have to navigate.** But mainly, they are a rare, elusive breed that you need for your business, and do not or cannot understand.

Oftentimes our CEO's will say, "I don't understand. I interviewed her three weeks ago, and now she is not available?" (Again...) *"Who does that?"* And I usually respond with, "Someone who needs to buy food to eat."

That is why we never stop hiring caregivers and placing them on our roster, because they need to pay bills NOW—not when you have a position for them. Now. Today!

What does that mean for you? *Play the odds.*

Great caregivers are always working for several agencies, so whoever has the best case/client/hours/pay usually wins. What that also means is, when you need them, they may be in between clients and be available to you. Since more than likely you have never depended on someone else's job performance to make you successful and build your reputation, I'd like to give a brief overview of how to treat those who truly will make or break you.

Like the Underground Railroad, caregivers work by word of mouth, so how you treat them and what your company environment and culture are like will be spread amongst the "Caregiver Community" faster than you can say, "You're Hired!"

Many companies have inside administrative staff that give off an attitude of arrogance to caregivers—that they are better than them. Many owners will talk down to them. I have also heard them described as a "Low Wage Work Force" and, although that is *relatively truthful*, it is not the most respectful term to use for those who are literally creating a safe and healthy environment for people they have never met.

✔ **Drop the arrogance and make sure that all of your office staff does, too.** I am willing to bet most CEO's aren't willing to go into an unfamiliar home, begin cleaning it up, take a stranger and change their clothes, their adult Depends, bathe them, feed them, and leave them with dignity and the care to make it through another day—all for $12-$15 per hour.

Low wage? Maybe. A better person than you? Definitely! And, in my company, they are treated as such. Great caregivers are like rare diamonds. They work and care for people because of their sensitivity and kindness, but when they are treated badly, that sensitivity can become surprisingly emotional or irrational, and that kindness can become aggressive, and sometimes it comes out of what you THINK is left field, but is actually from a lack of communication and listening that happens when people are treated as pawns.

"Caregivers...are a rare, elusive breed that you need for your business, and do not or cannot understand."

✔ **Put yourself in their shoes.** Imagine all day, every day, waiting on someone to give you a job, schedule, client, basically a paycheck. Now imagine that same person cancelling you because the client didn't come home from the hospital, went into the hospital, the daughter decided to care for the parent, the hours went from eight hours a day, five days a week, to four hours *twice* a week, and you're expected to stay and care for that client anyway?

~Imagine someone calling you at 9 p.m. asking you to cover a shift at 11 p.m.

~Imagine your kids need groceries and your rent needs to get paid, and someone is haggling with you over a mistake on your check?

~Imagine calling into the office with a complaint and not being listened to, then being told that it will be looked into and nothing changes.

~Imagine being offered a great job with a client that sounds like a dream only to find out this client has roaches, can't stand, or needs to be lifted and is 175 pounds.

~Imagine people telling you the client is "close by" and, after driving for an hour, you realize they are 30 miles from home and you are out of gas. And *then* imagine a staffer telling you that is not their problem.

~And after ALL of those things, imagine plastering a smile on your face and doing backbreaking work for someone else for $12-$15 per hour.

Stop asking or thinking that you can remain distant and "professional" and "manage" these special people.

Now, you can develop a structure for your business, which from the time we were three years old every person needs, and you can have boundaries and clear expectations—that is a necessity. But remember what you are asking them to do for you each and every time, and you will be amazed at the loyalty, *and heart*, of this incredible "Low Wage" workforce.

Like any numbers game, for every 10 hired, you will find one spectacular caregiver, two good caregivers, three caregivers that will work for you but don't really have it all together, and four who just don't work out. So the rule is, for every 10 you hire, you truly get *six*, and where they each will fall in the good, great, terrible, unavailable spectrum is always an anomaly.

"Great caregivers are always working for several agencies, so whoever has the best case/client/hours/pay usually wins. What that also means is, when you need them, they may be in between clients and be available to you."

✔ **Quickly get rid of bad apples.** We call it: *"No Call, No Show, No Job. No Second Chances."*

Also, if you have more than two complaints of the same type (late, rude, lazy, lack of client care), then more than likely you have a third string caregiver, which means that he or she can literally be placed as a fill in for one day, and then you have to keep moving her/him. So you may as well have "The Talk," along with a written warning, and then be prepared to let them go if a third complaint arises.

The same way there are some Caregiving Angels, there are also some Caregiving Nightmares, and you cannot afford to allow them into the population we serve. They belong anywhere else but in the home of a vulnerable person who has entrusted YOU with their very life.

THE BOTTOM LINE

Have a Mission, Vision and Company Culture that rests on Service First.

Have Integrity in your Care. Make sure you have many community partners to refer to and work with.

Be the Expert, drive the conversation with clients and be honest about Care Needs.

Treat your workforce well, with kindness and respect for the job they do, and quickly excise those that don't represent your brand.

Remember to have fun! Home care is a long-term, continually-changing career or business choice that is cyclical and challenging in nature, and not for the weak, so kindness and compassion are always the best medicine.

~~~

I wish you well on your journey. Feel free to reach out for consulting, or to buy into one of our franchise systems, or just to say hi:

L.smith.pratt@gmail.com

Your Care Is My Business.

The Home Care Bible

ABOUT THE AUTHOR

Lia Smith-Pratt began her career in home care as a Caregiver and CNA, working for private duty agencies and skilled care facilities over 30 years ago. She then moved into Home Care by working as a staffing director; subsequently managing two large home care agencies. Ms. Smith-Pratt began to see a trend in management and mindset that was not conducive to establishing quality care of the Seniors who were the primary clients, or of the caregivers who cared for them.

In April of 2000, she started her own agency, A Better Solution In Home Care, Inc. At the time of this publication, Ms. Smith-Pratt has been in business for over 18 years, learning from mistakes and adjusting her philosophies along the way. As a result, she has slowly raised her brand name within the industry, creating a thriving and well-known Home Care agency.

Ms. Smith-Pratt recently added Skilled Nursing Care and Medicare Certified Home Health to her Service Structure, and also offers Placement Services, all of which has increased her company's reputation and revenue streams while better serving the Senior/Home Care community. In 2015, Ms. Smith-Pratt took on a Partner and began to franchise her Agency Concept.

This book is a culmination of both the winning strategies and missteps that she has seen not only her

"Baby CEO's" make—but also owners all over the country, when trying to establish themselves in the industry. Making this book available to not just her Franchise Partners but to all home care owners is indicative of the drive and purpose of Lia Smith-Pratt, who is a fiercely competitive business woman. Ms. Smith-Pratt prefers to educate ALL home care owners in the Spirit of Service.

The tips she shares are helpful to owners who do not want to make costly mistakes, and who want to create financially successful agencies while maintaining an environment and company culture of *integrity* and *dedication* to the Seniors and Medically Fragile population in their care.

Other Books Written by L. Smith-Pratt: *Just Saying...1: Daily FB Reflections & Poetic Musings; Spiritual Lessons for My Daughters...Sisters...and Friends: Just Saying...2;* and *Smart Steps to Big Dreams: Life and Business Experiences to Consider.*

The Home Care Bible

READERS' NOTES:

The Home Care Bible

READERS' NOTES:

READERS' NOTES:

Made in the USA
Middletown, DE
22 January 2021